A
Pocket Manual
of
Differential
Diagnosis

P9-APB-323

A Pocket Manual of Differential Diagnosis

Stephen N. Adler, M.D.
Clinical Instructor, Department of Medicine,
University of Oklahoma College of Medicine,
Oklahoma City; Medical Director,
Respiratory Therapy, Mercy Health Center,
Oklahoma City

Mildred Lam, M.D.
Assistant Professor of Medicine, Nephrology Division,
Case Western Reserve University School of Medicine,
Cleveland; Metropolitan General Hospital, Cleveland

Alfred F. Connors, Jr., M.D.
Assistant Professor of Medicine, Pulmonary Division,
Case Western Reserve University School of Medicine,
Cleveland; Metropolitan General Hospital, Cleveland

Little, Brown and Company   Boston

Library of Congress Catalog Card No. 81-86044

ISBN 0-316-01106-1

Printed in the United States of America

DON

To our parents

Contents

Preface

Physicians frequently encounter symptoms, signs, and other data that require interpretation. The formulation of a complete differential diagnosis is essential to the correct interpretation of clinical data. The main difficulty in compiling a complete differential diagnosis is that physicians cannot remember everything. While they may intend to "look it up," too often they do not because the information is located in multiple sources at the library or at home, not at the bedside. We felt that this information, brought together in one source and made available in pocket form, would be a valuable aid to clinicians, house staff, and medical students.

A Pocket Manual of Differential Diagnosis provides a guide to the differential diagnosis of over 200 symptoms, physical signs, and other abnormal findings. This book is small enough for the physician to carry in a coat pocket and use at the bedside. The entries have been chosen to be useful to clinicians caring primarily for adult patients in the United States.

The book consists of 12 sections, divided according to organ system and arranged in alphabetical order, plus a section on drugs, which is a compendium of tables offering information on selected drug therapy. Each organ-system section consists of entries of abnormal findings and their differential diagnoses. Within each section, the entries generally are arranged in the following order: symptoms, physical signs, laboratory findings, x-rays, and disease processes. Within each differential list, common entities usually precede uncommon ones. Although considerable effort was made to be comprehensive, we excluded entities with questionable documentation. After each entry, references are provided as sources for further reading. Cross-references make possible easy access to related topics. Finally, space has been provided after each entry and section for users' inevitable personal additions.

We are grateful to Hal Balyeat, M.D., Randy Eichner, M.D., Ronald Jantzen, M.D., Donald Landstrom, M.D., William McCreight, M.D., Thomas Murphy, M.D., Ronald Painton, M.D., Hanna Saadah, M.D., and Galen Robbins, M.D., for their helpful suggestions and criticism. We would also like to thank Carol Snarey of Little, Brown for her patience and hard work. We extend special thanks to Solomon Papper, M.D., Distinguished Professor and Head, Department of Medicine, University of Oklahoma College of Medicine, for his encouragement and support.

S. N. A.
M. L.
A. F. C.

A
Pocket Manual
of
Differential
Diagnosis

1
Acid-Base and Electrolyte Disorders

1-A. Acid-Base Nomogram*

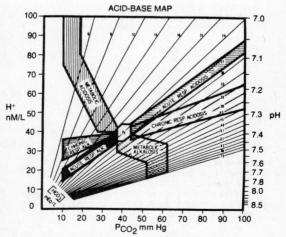

*From Goldberg M, Green SB, Moss ML, et al: Computer-Based Instruction and Diagnosis of Acid-Base Disorders. *JAMA* 223:270, 1973. Copyright © 1973 by the American Medical Association.

1-B. Metabolic Acidosis

Increased Anion Gap
Uremia
Ketoacidosis
  Diabetic
  Alcoholic
  Starvation
Lactic acidosis (see 1-E)
Toxins
  Aspirin
  Methanol
  Ethylene glycol
  Paraldehyde
Nonketotic hyperosmolar coma
Inborn errors of metabolism (e.g., maple syrup urine disease, methylmalonic aciduria)

Normal Anion Gap
Gastrointestinal loss .
  Diarrhea
  Ileal loop, ureterosigmoidostomy
  Small-bowel or pancreatic fistula or drainage
  Anion-exchange resin (e.g., cholestyramine)
Renal loss
  Renal tubular acidosis
  Hypoaldosteronism
  Carbonic anhydrase inhibitors
  Tubulointerstitial renal disease
  Urinary tract obstruction
Acidifying agents (e.g., ammonium chloride, arginine hydrochloride, lysine hydrochloride
Sulfur ingestion
Hyperalimentation with excess of cationic amino acids
Dilutional acidosis

References
1. Cohen JJ, Kassirer JP: Acid-Base Metabolism. In general reference 7, p 181.
2. Kaehny WD, Gabow PA: Pathogenesis and Management of Metabolic Acidosis and Alkalosis. In general reference 17, p 115.

1-C. Respiratory Acidosis*

Neuromuscular Causes
Brain stem or high-spinal-cord injury
Ingestion or overdose (tranquilizers, sedatives, anes-
    thetics, anticholinesterases)
Primary hypoventilation
Sleep apnea syndromes
Guillain-Barré syndrome
Myasthenia gravis
Poliomyelitis
Botulism
Diaphragmatic paralysis
Primary myopathy involving respiratory muscles

Airway Obstruction
Upper airway
    Laryngeal
    Tracheal
    Obstructive sleep apnea
Lower airway
    Mechanical
        Foreign body
        Neoplasm
    Bronchospasm
        Acute
        Chronic

Cardiopulmonary-Thoracic Causes
Cardiac arrest
Severe pneumonia
Severe pulmonary edema
Massive pulmonary embolus
Smoke inhalation
Pneumothorax
Restrictive disease of thorax (e.g., scleroderma, kypho-
    scoliosis)
Chest trauma

References
1. Cohen JJ, Kassirer JP: Acid-Base Metabolism. In general reference 7, p 181.
2. Kaehny WD: Pathogenesis and Management of Respiratory and Mixed Acid-Base Disorders. In general
   reference 17, p 159.

*See also 13-M.

1-D. Anion Gap

Increased
Without acidosis
    Administration of sodium salts of unmeasured anions
        (e.g., citrate, lactate, acetate)
    High-dose penicillin or carbenicillin
    Respiratory or metabolic alkalosis
    Dehydration
With acidosis
    Uremia
    Ketoacidosis
        Diabetic
        Starvation
        Alcoholic
    Nonketotic hyperosmolar coma
    Lactic acidosis (see 1-E)
    Toxins
        Aspirin
        Methanol
        Ethylene glycol
        Paraldehyde
    Inborn errors of metabolism

Decreased
Dilution
Hypoalbuminemia
Hypernatremia, severe
Hyperviscosity
Bromism
Paraproteinemia
Hypercalcemia, hypermagnesemia
Lithium toxicity

References
1. Emmett M, Narins RG: Clinical Use of the Anion Gap.
   Medicine 56:38, 1977.
2. Oh MS, Carroll HJ: Current Concepts: The Anion Gap.
   N Engl J Med 297:814, 1977.

1-E. Lactic Acidosis

Increased oxygen demand
   Excessive exercise
   Prolonged generalized seizures
Decreased oxygen delivery
   Cardiac arrest
   Shock
   Severe anemia
   Severe hypoxia
   Cardiopulmonary bypass
Liver failure
Alcohol intoxication
Glycogen storage disease
Diabetes mellitus (severe ketoacidosis)
Leukemia, lymphoma
Chronic renal failure
Pancreatitis
Pregnancy
Phenformin
Isoniazid overdose
Iron intoxication
Idiopathic

References
1. Kaehny WD, Gabow PA: Pathogenesis and Management of Metabolic Acidosis and Alkalosis. In general reference 17, p 115.
2. Cohen JJ, Kassirer JP: Acid-Base Metabolism. In general reference 7, p 181.
3. Kreisberg RA: Lactate Homeostasis and Lactic Acidosis. *Ann Intern Med* 92:227 1980

1-F. Metabolic Alkalosis

Chloride-Responsive (Urine Cl^- < 20 mEq/L)
Vomiting, nasogastric suction
Diuretics
Chloride diarrhea
Villous adenoma
Cystic fibrosis
Posthypercapnia

Chloride-Resistant (Urine Cl^- > 20 mEq/L)
Primary or secondary aldosteronism
Cushing's syndrome, ectopic ACTH
Bartter's syndrome
Licorice ingestion
Excessive use of chewing tobacco
Severe potassium depletion

Miscellaneous
Alkalinizing agents (e.g., bicarbonate, citrate, lactate)
Milk-alkali syndrome
Hypoparathyroidism
Massive transfusion
Nonparathyroid hypercalcemia (e.g., secondary to bony
    metastases, multiple myeloma)
Glucose ingestion after starvation
Carbenicillin, penicillin (massive doses)

References
1. Kaehny WD, Gabow PA: Pathogenesis and Management of Metabolic Acidosis and Alkalosis. In general reference 17, p 115.
2. Kassirer JP: Current Concepts: Serious Acid-Base Disorders. *N Engl J Med* 291:773, 1974.

1-G. Respiratory Alkalosis

Central Causes
Anxiety
Aspirin toxicity
Fever
Hypoxia
Head trauma
Brain tumor
Central nervous system infection
Cerebrovascular accident

Pulmonary Causes
Pneumonia
Pulmonary embolus
Interstitial lung disease
Adult respiratory distress syndrome
Congestive heart failure
Altitude

Other
Hepatic insufficiency
Shock (especially gram-negative sepsis)
Mechanical ventilation

References
1. Cohen JJ, Kassirer JP: Acid-Base Metabolism. In general reference 7, p 181.
2. Kaehny WD: Pathogenesis and Management of Respiratory and Mixed Acid-Base Disorders. In general reference 17, p 159.

1-H. Hypernatremia

Pure Water Loss
Inability to obtain water (e.g., coma, dementia, infancy)
Inability to swallow
Impaired thirst drive (e.g., hypothalamic lesion)
Increased insensible loss

Excessive Sodium Intake
Substitution of salt for sugar in infant formula
Seawater ingestion
Iatrogenic sodium administration
  Sodium bicarbonate (cardiac arrest, treatment of lactic
    acidosis)
  Hypertonic saline (therapeutic abortion)
Mineralocorticoid or glucocorticoid excess
  Primary aldosteronism
  Cushing's syndrome
  Ectopic ACTH production

Loss of Water in Excess of Sodium
(Without Concomitant Water Intake)
Gastrointestinal loss (e.g., vomiting, diarrhea, intestinal
    fistula)
Skin loss (e.g., burns, sweating)
Renal loss
  Osmotic diuresis
    Infant formula (especially cow's milk)
    Tube feedings
    Mannitol
    Diabetic ketoacidosis
    Chronic renal failure with salt wasting
    Partial urinary tract obstruction, postobstructive
      diuresis
    Diuretic phase of acute renal failure
  Excessive use of diuretics
  Diabetes insipidus
    Central
    Nephrogenic
      Congenital
      Hypokalemia
      Hypercalcemia
      Drugs (see below)
  Drugs
    Lithium
    Demeclocycline
    Alcohol

　　Phenytoin
　　Propoxyphene
　　Amphotericin B
　　Methoxyflurane
　　Colchicine
　　Vinblastine
Peritoneal dialysis

Essential Hypernatremia (Reset Osmostat)

Reference
1. Ross EJ, Christie SBM: Hypernatremia. *Medicine* 48:441, 1969.

1-I. Hyponatremia

States with Decreased Extracellular Fluid Volume
Gastrointestinal loss (e.g., vomiting, diarrhea)
Third-space loss (e.g., burns, sweating, hemorrhagic pancreatitis)
Renal loss
　Diuretic use
　Renal salt-wasting (e.g., advanced chronic renal failure, interstitial disease, renal tubular acidosis)
　Adrenal insufficiency

States with Increased Extracellular Fluid Volume
Congestive heart failure
Cirrhosis and ascites
Nephrotic syndrome
Psychogenic polydipsia with massive water intake (> 20–25 L/day)
Beer drinking (excessive) in association with malnutrition

States with Normal Extracellular Fluid Volume
Syndrome of inappropriate antidiuretic hormone (ADH)
　Central nervous system lesion, e.g.:
　　Tumor
　　Trauma
　　Encephalitis

    Meningitis
    Cerebrovascular accident
    Brain abscess
    Guillain-Barré syndrome
  Pulmonary disease, e.g.:
    Tumor
    Pneumonia
    Lung abscess
    Tuberculosis
  Carcinoma (especially lung, pancreas, duodenum)
  Porphyria
  Acute psychosis
  Hypothyroidism
  Postoperative state
  Pain
  Positive-pressure respiration
Drugs
  Nicotine
  Chlorpropamide
  Tolbutamide
  Phenformin
  Clofibrate
  Vincristine
  Cyclophosphamide
  Isoproterenol
  Morphine
  Barbiturates
  General anesthetics
  Indomethacin
  Carbamazepine
  Acetaminophen
  Diuretics
Essential (reset osmostat)

Reference

1. Schrier RW: Renal Sodium Excretion, Edematous Disorders, and Diuretic Use. In general reference 17, p 65.

1-J. Hyperkalemia

Pseudohyperkalemia
Use of tourniquet
Hemolysis (in vitro)
Leukocytosis, thrombocytosis

Intracellular-to-Extracellular K⁺ Shift
Acidosis
Hyperkalemic periodic paralysis
Digitalis intoxication

K⁺ Load (Especially in Presence of Renal Insufficiency)
K⁺ supplements
K⁺-rich foods
K⁺-containing salt substitute
Intravenous K⁺
Transfusion of aged blood
Hemolysis
K⁺-containing drugs (e.g., potassium penicillin)
Cell destruction postchemotherapy (especially with
    leukemia, lymphoma, myeloma)
Rhabdomyolysis
Extensive crush injury or tissue necrosis

Decreased K⁺ Excretion
Renal failure (acute or chronic)
K⁺-sparing diuretics
Aldosterone deficiency (e.g., adrenal insufficiency,
    hyporeninemic hypoaldosteronism)
Selective defect in renal K⁺ excretion
    Lupus erythematosus
    Sickle cell disease
    Obstructive uropathy
    Renal transplantation
    Congenital

References
1. Schultze RG, Nissenson AR: Potassium: Physiology
   and Pathophysiology. In general reference 7, p 113.
2. Gabow PA, Peterson LN: Disorders of Potassium
   Metabolism. In general reference 17, p 183.

1-K. Hypokalemia

Extracellular-to-intracellular K⁺ shifts
  Alkalosis
  Hypokalemic periodic paralysis
  Increased plasma insulin
Decreased intake
Geophagia
Gastrointestinal loss
  Fistula
  Vomiting, nasogastric suction
  Diarrhea, laxative or enema abuse
  Malabsorption
  Ureterosigmoidostomy, ileal loop
  Villous adenoma
Urinary loss
  Diuretic therapy
  Primary aldosteronism
  Secondary aldosteronism (especially malignant hypertension, renal artery stenosis, Bartter's syndrome, renal hemangiopericytoma)
  ACTH (secondary to pituitary or ectopic secretion)
  Adrenal hyperplasia
  Liddle's syndrome
  Excessive licorice ingestion
  Excessive use of chewing tobacco
  Renal tubular acidosis
  Diuresis during recovery from obstruction or acute renal failure
  Osmotic diuresis
  Carbenicillin, penicillin, amphotericin B
  Hypomagnesemia
  Interstitial nephritis
  Acute leukemia
  Familial

References
1. Schultze RG, Nissenson AR: Potassium: Physiology and Pathophysiology. In general reference 7, p 113.
2. Gabow P, Peterson LN: Disorders of Potassium Metabolism. In general reference 17, p 183.

1-L. Hypercalcemia

Hyperparathyroidism
  Primary
    Adenoma
    Hyperplasia
    Carcinoma
    Multiple endocrine adenomatosis
  Secondary
  Ectopic
Malignancy
  Bony metastases
  Humoral factors
    Parathyroid hormone (PTH)
    PTH-like substances
    Prostaglandins
    Osteoclast-activating factor
Vitamin D intoxication
Vitamin A intoxication
Sarcoidosis
Tuberculosis
Berylliosis
Hyperthyroidism
Adrenal insufficiency
Immobilization (in association with rapid bone turnover
    states, e.g., adolescence or Paget's disease)
Milk-alkali syndrome
Ion-exchange resins (e.g., cholestyramine)
Recovery from acute renal failure following rhab-
    domyolysis
Thiazide diuretics
Acromegaly
Hypophosphatasia
Hypophosphatemia
Idiopathic infantile hypercalcemia
Hypothyroidism in children
Blue-diaper syndrome
Familial hypocalciuric hypercalcemia
Metaphyseal chondrodysplasia

References
1. Parfitt AM, Kleerekoper M: Clinical Disorders of Calcium, Phosphorus, and Magnesium Metabolism. In
   general reference 7, p 947.
2. Popovtzer MM, Knochel JP: Disorders of Calcium,
   Phosphorus, Vitamin D, and Parathyroid Hormone Activity. In general reference 17, p 223.

1-M. Hypocalcemia

Vitamin D deficiency states
  Atmospheric or dietary deprivation
  Malabsorption (see 6-G)
    Postgastrectomy
    Sprue
    Pancreatic insufficiency
    Hepatobiliary disease with bile salt deficiency
    Laxative abuse
Abnormal metabolism of vitamin D
  Renal failure (acute and chronic)
  Liver failure
  Vitamin D–dependent rickets
  Anticonvulsants, microsomal enzyme inducers
Hypoparathyroidism
  Congenital
  Idiopathic (infantile and adolescent-onset types)
  Acquired
    Surgical
    Iron overload
    Irradiation
    Neoplasm
Pseudohypoparathyroidism
Magnesium depletion
Phosphate administration
  Enemas, laxatives
  Intravenous administration
  Cow's milk in infants
Malignancy
  Osteoblastic metastases (especially carcinoma of
    prostate, breast)
  Malignancy with increased thyrocalcitonin levels (espe-
    cially medullary carcinoma of thyroid)
Cytotoxic therapy for leukemia, lymphoma
Rhabdomyolysis
Acute pancreatitis
Agents causing decreased bone resorption (e.g., ac-
  tinomycin, calcitonin, mithramycin)
Calcium-complexing agents (e.g., citrate, EDTA)
Massive transfusion, plasma exchange
Healing phase of rickets, osteitis fibrosa, thyrotoxic os-
  teopathy
Hyperkalemic periodic paralysis, acute
Osteopetrosis
Neonatal tetany

References
1. Parfitt AM, Kleerekoper M: Clinical Disorders of Calcium, Phosphorus, and Magnesium Metabolism. In general reference 7, p 947.
2. Popovtzer MM, Knochel JP: Disorders of Calcium, Phosphorus, Vitamin D, and Parathyroid Hormone Activity. In general reference 17, p 223.

1-N. Hyperphosphatemia

Increased Renal Tubular Reabsorption
Hypoparathyroidism
Pseudohypoparathyroidism
Hyperthyroidism
Volume contraction
Fever
Juvenile hypogonadism
Postmenopausal state
Acromegaly
Tumoral calcinosis

Increased Load
Renal failure
Increased absorption (e.g., vitamin D intoxication)
Oral or intravenous phosphate
Phosphate-containing laxatives, enemas
Transfusion
Respiratory acidosis
Diabetic ketoacidosis
Lactic acidosis
Malignant hyperpyrexia
Rhabdomyolysis
Cytotoxic therapy
Hemolysis
Familial (rare)

Reference
1. Parfitt AM, Kleerekoper M: Clinical Disorders of Calcium, Phosphorus, and Magnesium Metabolism. In general reference 7, p 947.

1-O. Hypophosphatemia

Decreased Intake and Absorption,
Increased Nonrenal Loss
Phosphate-binding antacids
Starvation, cachexia
Vomiting
Diarrhea, malabsorption
Hemodialysis

Transcellular Shift
Carbohydrate load with or without insulin administration
Nutritional recovery syndrome
Alkalosis, especially respiratory
Androgens, anabolic steroids
Catecholamines
Sepsis
Heat stroke
Gout, acute
Aspirin poisoning
Pregnancy
Hypothyroidism
Myocardial infarction, acute

Renal Loss
Hyperparathyroidism, primary
Diuretics, especially thiazides
Volume expansion (including hyperaldosteronism)
Hypokalemia
Hypomagnesemia
Steroid therapy, Cushing's syndrome
Estrogens, oral contraceptives
Acidosis
Renal tubular defects (e.g., Fanconi's syndrome)
Genetic causes (e.g., vitamin D–resistant rickets)
Tumor phosphaturia (mesenchymoma, neurofibroma,
    pleomorphic sarcoma, sclerosing or cavernous
    hemangioma)
Recovery from prolonged hypothermia
Renal transplantation

Mixed Mechanisms
Alcoholism
Diabetic ketoacidosis
Liver disease
Hyperalimentation
Recovery from severe burns
Vitamin D deficiency

References
1. Parfitt AM, Kleerekoper M: Clinical Disorders of Calcium, Phosphorus, and Magnesium Metabolism. In general reference 7, p 947.
2. Fitzgerald FT: Hypophosphatemia. *Adv Intern Med* 23:137, 1978.

1-P. Hypermagnesemia

Renal failure
Increased magnesium load (especially in presence of renal insufficiency)
  Catabolic states
  Diabetic ketoacidosis
  Magnesium-containing laxatives or antacids
  Treatment of eclampsia (mother and infant)
Increased renal magnesium reabsorption
  Hyperparathyroidism
  Familial hypocalciuric hypercalcemia
  Hypothyroidism
  Mineralocorticoid deficiency, Addison's disease

References
1. Parfitt AM, Kleerekoper M: Clinical Disorders of Calcium, Phosphorus, and Magnesium Metabolism. In general reference 7, p 947.
2. Alfrey AC: Disorders of Magnesium Metabolism. In general reference 17, p 299.

1-Q. Hypomagnesemia

Redistribution
Postparathyroidectomy
Refeeding after starvation
Correction of metabolic acidosis
Intravenous glucose, hyperalimentation
Acute pancreatitis

Decreased Intake, Increased Extrarenal Loss
Malnutrition
Alcoholism
Diarrhea, malabsorption (especially involving distal ileum)
Nasogastric suction
Biliary fistula
Sweating, burns
Lactation
Dialysis

Increased Renal Loss
Saline or osmotic diuresis
Postobstructive or post-acute-renal-failure diuresis
Diuretics
Diabetic ketoacidosis
Alcohol abuse
Carbohydrate load
Ammonium chloride
Tubulointerstitial renal disease
Aminoglycoside nephrotoxicity
Hypercalciuria
Vitamin D therapy
Primary or secondary aldosteronism
Bartter's syndrome
Potassium depletion
Hypoparathyroidism
Hyperthyroidism
Inappropriate ADH secretion
Renal transplantation
Familial
Idiopathic

References
1. Parfitt AM, Kleerekoper M: Clinical Disorders of Calcium, Phosphorus, and Magnesium Metabolism. In general reference 7, p 947.
2. Alfrey AC: Disorders of Magnesium Metabolism. In general reference 17, p 299.

2
Cardiovascular System

2-A. Chest Pain

Skin and subcutaneous lesions (including adiposis
    dolorosa, thrombophlebitis of thoracoepigastric vein
    [Mondor's disease])
Breast lesions
    Fibroadenosis
    Chronic cystic mastitis
    Acute breast abscess or mastitis
    Carcinoma
Musculoskeletal disorders
    Bruised or fractured rib
    Periostitis
    Periosteal hematoma
    Costochondritis (Tietze's syndrome)
    Slipping costal cartilage
    Intercostal muscle "stitch" or cramp
    Intercostal myositis
    Pectoral or other muscular strain
    Shoulder girdle disorders
    Cervical disk herniation
    Thoracic outlet syndromes
Neuralgia
    Herpes zoster
    Tabes dorsalis
    Neurofibroma

Pericardial disease
  Pericarditis (see 2-I)
  Neoplasm
  Congenital absence of left pericardium
Mediastinal disease
  Mediastinal emphysema
  Neoplasm
  Mediastinitis
Cardiovascular disease
  Acute myocardial infarction
  Angina pectoris
  Aortic valvular disease
  Idiopathic hypertrophic subaortic stenosis (IHSS)
  Mitral valve prolapse
  Acute aortic dissection
  Thoracic aortic aneurysm
  Myocarditis
  Primary pulmonary hypertension
  Ruptured sinus of Valsalva aneurysm
Pleural or pulmonary disease
  Pleuritis of any etiology (see 13-F)
  Tracheobronchitis
  Pneumonia
  Pulmonary thromboembolism
  Neoplasm
    Bronchogenic carcinoma
    Metastatic tumor
    Mesothelioma
  Other parenchymal lesions
Gastrointestinal disease
  Esophageal lesions
    Esophagitis
    Esophageal spasm
    Mallory-Weiss syndrome
    Esophageal rupture
    Foreign body
    Carcinoma
    Zenker's diverticulum
    Plummer-Vinson syndrome
  Peptic ulcer disease (with or without perforation)
  Biliary disease
    Acute cholecystitis
    Biliary colic
  Pancreatitis
  Subphrenic abscess
  Splenic infarct
Thyroiditis
Psychogenic causes

References
1. General reference 5, p 224.
2. Braunwald E: Chest Pain and Palpitation. In general reference 1, p 28.

2-B. Edema

Localized
Venous or lymphatic obstruction
  Venous thrombosis
  Tumor invasion or compression (e.g., superior vena cava syndrome)
  Surgical or radiation damage
  Filariasis
Inflammatory disease
Allergic process
Physical or chemical trauma
Stings and bites
Immobilized or paralyzed limb
Congenital lymphedema

Generalized
Biventricular congestive heart failure
Cor pulmonale
Pericardial disease
  Chronic constrictive pericarditis
  Pericardial effusion
Hepatic cirrhosis
Hypoalbuminemic states
  Nephrotic syndrome
  Protein-losing enteropathy
  Malnutrition
  Severe chronic disease
Acute and chronic renal failure with volume overload
Inferior vena cava obstruction
Myxedema
Iatrogenic salt overload
  Enteral feeding
  Intravenous fluid administration

Drugs
    Carbenicillin
    Phenylbutazone
    Indomethacin
    Corticosteroids
    Hydralazine
    Guanethidine
    Diazoxide
    Minoxidil
Trichinosis
Idiopathic cyclic edema
Hereditary angioneurotic edema

Reference
1. Braunwald E: Edema. In general reference 1, p 171.

2-C. Palpitation*

Palpitation without Arrhythmia
Noncardiac disorders
    Anxiety
    Exercise
    Anemia
    Fever
    Volume depletion
    Thyrotoxicosis
    Menopausal syndrome
    Hypoglycemia
    Pheochromocytoma
    Aortic aneurysm
    Migraine syndrome
    Arteriovenous fistula
    Diaphragmatic flutter
    Drugs
        Sympathomimetic agents
        Ganglionic blockers
        Digitalis
        Nitrates
        Aminophylline

    Atropine
    Coffee, tea
    Tobacco
    Alcohol
    Thyroid extract
Cardiac disorders
  Aortic regurgitation
  Aortic stenosis
  Patent ductus arteriosus
  Ventricular septal defect
  Atrial septal defect
  Marked cardiomegaly
  Acute left ventricular failure
  Hyperkinetic heart syndrome
  Tricuspid insufficiency
  Pericarditis
  Prosthetic heart valve
  Electronic pacemaker

Palpitation with Arrhythmia†
Extrasystoles
Bradyarrhythmias
Tachyarrhythmias

Reference
1. Braunwald E: Chest Pain and Palpitation. In general reference 1, p 28.

---

*Palpitation is the sensation of disturbed heartbeat. This entry was modified from Shander D: Palpitation and Disorders of the Heartbeat. In Friedman HH (Ed): *Problem-Oriented Medical Diagnosis* (2nd ed). Boston: Little, Brown, 1977.
†See 2-O.

2-D. Hypertension*

Systolic and Diastolic
Pseudohypertension (e.g., wrong-sized cuff)
Primary (essential)
Renal causes
  Parenchymal
  Vascular
  Renoprival (following bilateral nephrectomy)
  Renin-producing tumor
  Liddle's syndrome
Endocrine causes
  Acromegaly
  Hypothyroidism
  Hypercalcemia
  Adrenal causes
    Congenital adrenal hyperplasia
    Cushing's syndrome
    Primary aldosteronism
    Pheochromocytoma
  Extraadrenal chromaffin tumors
  Exogenous
    Estrogens
    Glucocorticoids
    Mineralocorticoids (e.g., licorice)
    Sympathomimetic agents
    Tyramine-containing foods and MAO inhibitors
Coarctation of aorta
Pregnancy-induced
Neurogenic causes
  Increased intracranial pressure
  Postoperative state
  Acute porphyria
  Lead poisoning
  Quadriplegia
  Diencephalic syndrome
  Familial dysautonomia
Increased intravascular volume
  Polycythemia vera
  Iatrogenic causes
Burns
Sleep apnea
Psychogenic causes

Systolic
Increased cardiac output and/or stroke volume
  Aortic valvular regurgitation

Arteriovenous fistula, patent ductus
Paget's disease
Beriberi
Thyrotoxicosis (endogenous or exogenous)
Anemia
Hyperkinetic circulation
Anxiety
Complete heart block
Aortic rigidity

References

1. Kaplan NM: Systemic Hypertension: Mechanisms and Diagnosis. In general reference 8, p 852.
2. Williams GH, Jagger PI, Braunwald E: Hypertensive Vascular Disease. In general reference 1, p 1167.

*Modified from Kaplan NM: Systemic Hypertension: Mechanisms and Diagnosis. In general reference 8, p 881.

2-E. Jugular Venous Distention

Extrathoracic Causes

Local venous obstruction of any cause (e.g., cervical goiter)
Circulatory overload of noncardiac etiology

Intrathoracic Causes

Valsalva maneuver
Retrosternal goiter
Superior vena cava syndrome
  Benign
  Malignant
Pericardial disease (see 2-I, 2-J)
  Cardiac tamponade
  Constrictive pericarditis
Cardiac disease
  Right heart failure of any etiology (see 2-G)

Restrictive cardiomyopathy
Right atrial myxoma
Hyperkinetic heart circulatory states
Pleuropulmonary disease
Pulmonary hypertension of any etiology (see 13-P)
Bronchial asthma
Chronic bronchitis and emphysema
Tension pneumothorax

References
1. General reference 5, p 389.
2. Friedman HH: Jugular Venous Pulse. In general reference 4, p 46.

2-F. Heart Murmurs*

Systolic
Early systolic
Physiologic (innocent)
Small ventricular septal defect
Large ventricular septal defect with pulmonary hypertension
Severe acute mitral regurgitation
Tricuspid regurgitation without pulmonary hypertension
Midsystolic
Physiologic (innocent)
Vibratory murmur
Pulmonary ejection murmur
Aortic ejection murmur of old age
Obstruction to left ventricular outflow
Valvular aortic stenosis
Fibrous subaortic stenosis
Supravalvular aortic stenosis
Idiopathic hypertrophic subaortic stenosis
Aortic valve prosthesis
Aortic dilatation
Transmitted murmur of mitral regurgitation
Aortic flow murmur in aortic regurgitation
Coarctation of aorta

*See also 2-N.

Supraclavicular arterial bruit
Obstruction to right ventricular outflow
  Pulmonic valvular stenosis
  Subpulmonic (infundibular) stenosis
Flow murmur of atrial septal defect
Idiopathic dilatation of pulmonary artery
Pulmonary hypertension of any cause (occasionally)
Late systolic
  Mitral valve prolapse
  Tricuspid valve prolapse
Holosystolic
  Mitral regurgitation
  Tricuspid regurgitation secondary to pulmonary hypertension
  Ventricular septal defect
  Patent ductus arteriosus with pulmonary hypertension

Diastolic

Early diastolic
  Aortic regurgitation
  Pulmonic regurgitation associated with pulmonary
    hypertension
Middiastolic
  Mitral stenosis
  Mitral valve prosthesis
  Tricuspid stenosis
  Atrial myxoma
  Left atrial ball-valve thrombus
  Austin Flint murmur
  Increased diastolic atrioventricular flow
    Mitral and tricuspid regurgitation
    Left-to-right shunt (e.g., ventricular septal defect)
    Acute rheumatic valvulitis
  Coronary artery stenosis
Presystolic
  Mitral stenosis
  Tricuspid stenosis
  Atrial myxoma
  Left-to-right shunt
  Complete heart block
  Severe pulmonic stenosis
  Fourth heart sound

Continuous

Pseudomurmur (e.g., pericardial friction rub)
Traumatic arteriovenous fistula
Patent ductus arteriosus
Surgically created aorticopulmonary fistula

Aorticopulmonary window without severe pulmonary
hypertension
Pulmonary embolism
Coronary arteriovenous fistula
Ruptured sinus of Valsalva aneurysm
Coarctation of aorta
Bronchial artery collateral circulation
Lutembacher's syndrome
Cervical venous hum
Mammary souffle

References
1. Craige E: Echophonocardiography and Other Non-
   invasive Techniques to Elucidate Heart Murmurs and
   to Solve Diagnostic Problems. In general reference 8, p
   70.
2. O'Rourke RA, Braunwald E: Physical Examination of
   the Heart. In general reference 1, p 993.
3. Shander D: Cardiovascular Problems: Palpitation and
   Disorders of the Heartbeat. In general reference 4, p
   100.

2-G. Congestive Heart Failure

Left Heart Failure
Hypertensive heart disease
Coronary artery disease
Acute myocardial infarction
Aortic and mitral valvular disease
Cardiomyopathy
Arrhythmias
Congenital heart disease
Endocarditis
Cardiotoxic drugs (e.g., Adriamycin)
Myocarditis
Acute rheumatic fever

Traumatic heart disease
Thyrotoxicosis
Thiamine deficiency
Anemia
Arteriovenous fistula (e.g., Paget's disease)
Neoplastic heart disease
Toxic shock syndrome
Pulmonary thromboembolism
Postcardioversion

Right Heart Failure (see 13-P)
Associated with pulmonary venous hypertension (post-capillary)
  Cardiac disease (see above)
  Pulmonary venous disease
    Mediastinal neoplasm or granuloma
    Mediastinitis
    Anomalous pulmonary venous return
    Congenital pulmonary venous stenosis
    Idiopathic pulmonary veno-occlusive disease
Associated with pulmonary arterial hypertension (pre-capillary)
  Lung and pleural disease
    Chronic bronchitis and emphysema
    Granulomatous disease (e.g., sarcoidosis)
    Fibrotic disease
    Neoplasm
    Chronic suppurative disease
    Collagen-vascular disease
    Other restrictive processes (see 13-O)
    Following lung resection
    Fibrothorax
    Chest wall deformity
      Kyphoscoliosis
      Thoracoplasty
  Alveolar hypoventilation
    Neuromuscular
    Primary alveolar hypoventilation
    Obesity
    Sleep apnea syndrome
    High-altitude pulmonary hypertension
  Intracardiac disease
    Increased flow associated with large left-to-right shunt
      Patent ductus arteriosus
      Atrial septal defect
      Ventricular septal defect
      Sinus of Valsalva aneurysm

Decreased flow
  Tetralogy of Fallot
  Peripheral pulmonary artery stenosis (or stenoses)
  Unilateral absence or stenosis of pulmonary artery
Vascular disease
  Pulmonary thromboembolic disease
    Thrombotic
    Septic
    Fat
    Air
    Amniotic fluid, trophoblastic
    Foreign material (e.g., talc)
    Parasitic
    Metastatic neoplasm
    Thrombosis associated with SS and SC hemoglobin
    Thrombosis associated with eclampsia
  Pulmonary arteritis
    Raynaud's disease
    Scleroderma
    CRST syndrome
    Schistosomiasis
    Rheumatoid arthritis
    Systemic lupus erythematosus
    Polymyositis, dermatomyositis
    Granulomatous arteritis
    Takayasu's disease
Without pulmonary hypertension
  Pulmonic stenosis
  Tricuspid stenosis (nonrheumatic)
  Tricuspid regurgitation not associated with pulmonary hypertension
  Decreased right ventricular compliance
  Ebstein's anomaly

References

1. General reference 26, p 1203.
2. Moser KM (Ed): *Pulmonary Vascular Diseases*. New York: Marcel Dekker, Inc., 1979.
3. Grossman W, Braunwald E: Pulmonary Hypertension. In general reference 8, p 835.

2-H. Cardiomyopathy

Congestive
Congenital
  Diabetes
  Familial
  Duchenne's muscular dystrophy
  Limb-girdle muscular dystrophy
  Myotonic dystrophy
  Refsum's disease
  Glycogen storage disorders
  Mucopolysaccharidoses
  Fabry's disease
  Gaucher's disease
Acquired
  Idiopathic
  Alcoholism
  Myocarditis
  Peripartum
  Uremia
  Obesity
  Sarcoidosis
  Hyperthermia
  Hypothermia
  Irradiation
  Acromegaly
  Hypophosphatemia
  Hypocalcemia
  Hemochromatosis
  Polymyositis, dermatomyositis
  Whipple's disease
  Amyloidosis
  Scleroderma
  Hypoxia
  Neoplasm
  Becker's disease
  Nutritional deficiency (e.g., thiamine)
  Endomyocardial fibrosis
  Toxins, drugs
    Daunorubicin
    Doxorubicin (Adriamycin)
    Cyclophosphamide
    Phosphate (poisoning)
    Phenothiazines
    Lithium
    Carbon monoxide
    Emetine

Chloroquine
Acetaminophen
Lead
Arsenic
Hydrocarbons
Antimony
Cobalt

Restrictive
Pseudocardiomyopathy (i.e., constrictive pericarditis)
Amyloidosis
Hemochromatosis
Sarcoidosis
Scleroderma
Neoplasm
Endocardial fibroelastosis
Loeffler's fibroplastic endocarditis
Endomyocardial fibrosis

Hypertrophic
Idiopathic hypertrophic subaortic stenosis (IHSS)
Glycogen storage disease (Pompe's disease)
Friedreich's ataxia

References
1. Wynne J, Braunwald E: The Cardiomyopathies and Myocarditides. In general reference 8, p 1437.
2. Goodwin JF: Congestive and Hypertrophic Cardiomyopathies: A Decade of Study. *Lancet* 1:731, 1970.

2-I. Pericarditis*

Idiopathic†
Infection
  Viral†
    Bacterial†
    Mycobacterial†
    Mycoplasmal
    Fungal†
    Parasitic†

*See also 2-J.

Acute myocardial infarction
Uremia†
Neoplasm†
Aortic dissection with hemopericardium
Connective-tissue or hypersensitivity diseases
    Post–myocardial infarction (Dressler's syndrome)
    Postpericardiectomy†
    Drugs
        Penicillin
        Isoniazid
        Methysergide
        Daunorubicin
        Emetine
    Systemic lupus erythematosus†
        Idiopathic
        Drug-related (e.g., hydralazine, procainamide)
    Mixed connective-tissue disease
    Scleroderma
    Rheumatoid arthritis†
    Polyarteritis nodosa†
    Polymyositis
    Reiter's syndrome
    Serum sickness
    Acute rheumatic fever
Traumatic†
    Penetrating wounds
    Catheter-induced cardiac perforation
    Blunt chest trauma
    Cardiopulmonary resuscitation
    Cardioversion
Noninfectious granulomatous diseases
    Cholesterol
        Idiopathic
        Rheumatoid arthritis
        Hypercholesterolemia
    Iatrogenic
        Talc or other foreign substance
    Sarcoidosis
    Wegener's granulomatosis
Postirradiation†
Esophageal rupture
Uncommon miscellaneous etiologies
    Congenital heart disease (e.g., atrial septal defect)
    Familial Mediterranean fever
    Right atrial myxoma

†May be associated with development of constrictive pericarditis.

Severe chronic anemia (e.g., thalassemia)
Pancreatitis
Whipple's disease
Acute gouty arthritis
Pulmonary thromboembolism
Takayasu's disease
Mulibrey nanism†

References
1. Darsee JR, Braunwald E: Diseases of the Pericardium. In general reference 8, p 1517.
2. Roberts WC, Spray TL: Pericardial Heart Disease. *Curr Probl Cardiol*, 1977, p 55.

2-J. Pericardial Effusion

Pericarditis (see 2-I)
Congestive heart failure
Hypoalbuminemia
Acute pancreatitis*
Chylopericardium*
Hemopericardium§
Myxedema*

References
1. Darsee JR, Braunwald E: Diseases of the Pericardium. In general reference 8, p 1517.
2. Roberts WC, Spray TL: Pericardial Heart Disease. *Curr Probl Cardiol*, 1977, p 55.

*May be associated with chronic constrictive pericarditis.
§May be associated with acute cardiac tamponade.

2-K. Hypotension and Shock

Hypoxia of any cause
Severe acidosis or alkalosis
Hypovolemia
  External losses
    Hemorrhage
    Gastrointestinal loss
    Renal loss (e.g., diuretic use)
    Cutaneous loss
      Burns
      Exudative lesions
      Perspiration and insensible loss without replacement
  Internal losses
    Hemorrhage (e.g., anticoagulant therapy)
      Hemothorax
      Hemoperitoneum
      Retroperitoneal hemorrhage
      Fracture
    Fluid sequestration
      Ascites
      Bowel obstruction
      Peritonitis
      Phlegmon (e.g., pancreatitis)
Infection
  Septicemia
  Specific infections (e.g., dengue fever)
  Toxic shock syndrome
Anaphylaxis
Endocrine disease
  Adrenal insufficiency
  Hypocalcemia or hypercalcemia
  Myxedema or thyroid storm
  Pheochromocytoma
  Pituitary failure
Cardiogenic causes
  Arrhythmia (see 2-O)
  Regurgitant lesions
    Acute mitral or aortic regurgitation
    Rupture of interventricular septum
    Giant left ventricular aneurysm
  Obstructive lesions
    Valvular stenosis
    Hypertrophic cardiomyopathy
    Atrial myxoma
    Intracardiac thrombus

Myopathy
  Acute myocardial infarction
  Congestive or restrictive cardiomyopathy
  Other myocardial disorders (associated with low cardiac output)
Pericardial disease
  Cardiac tamponade
  Constrictive pericarditis
Aortic lesions
  Acute dissection
  Coarctation
  Rupture (e.g., trauma or aneurysm)
Pleuropulmonary disease
  Tension pneumothorax
  Pulmonary thromboembolism (including amniotic fluid, air, tumor embolus)
  Primary pulmonary hypertension
  Eisenmenger reaction
Hypothermia and hyperthermia
Drugs and toxins
  Drug overdose and poisoning (e.g., barbiturates)
  Antihypertensive agents
  Other vasodilators (e.g., nitroglycerin)
  Heavy metals
Neuropathic causes
  Brain stem failure
  Spinal cord dysfunction
  Autonomic insufficiency

References

1. Engelman K, Braunwald E: Hypotension and the Shock Syndrome. In general reference 1, p 175.
2. Sobel BE: Cardiac and Non-cardiac Forms of Acute Circulatory Collapse (Shock). In general reference 8, p 590.

2-L. Cardiac Arrest
(Sudden Cardiopulmonary Collapse)

Arrhythmia (with or without digitalis intoxication)
    Tachyarrhythmia
        Ventricular fibrillation
        Ventricular tachycardia
        Supraventricular tachycardias
    Bradyarrhythmias
        Sinus bradycardia
        Junctional rhythm
        Atrioventricular block
        Idioventricular rhythm
    Asystole
Upper airway obstruction
Acute respiratory failure with hypoxemia and/or hyper-
    carbia
Hypoxia of any cause (e.g., carbon monoxide poisoning)
Severe acidosis or alkalosis
Hypoglycemia
Addisonian crisis
Drug overdose, allergy, or adverse reaction; e.g.:
    Narcotics
    Insulin
    Sedatives
    Quinidine
    Nitrates
    Aminophylline
    Propranolol
    Warfarin
    Penicillins
    Sulfonamides
    Antihypertensive agents
Shock of any etiology (see also 2-K), especially:
    Hypovolemia
    Tension pneumothorax
    Cardiac tamponade
    Anaphylaxis
    Sepsis
    Aortic dissection
    Pulmonary embolism (of any type)
    Acute myocardial infarction
    Other cardiac causes
        Valvular disease (e.g., aortic stenosis)
        Myocarditis
        Cardiac rupture
        Mitral valve prolapse

Electrolyte abnormality (especially potassium, calcium,
      magnesium)
Hypothermia or hyperthermia
Electric shock
Insect stings and bites
Neurologic disorders
   Stroke
   Seizure
   Brain stem compression of any cause
   Infection
Sudden infant death syndrome

References

1. Lown B: Cardiovascular Collapse and Sudden Cardiac
   Death. In general reference 8, p 778.
2. Spivak JL: Cardiac Arrest and Resuscitation. In JL
   Spivak and HV Barnes (Eds): *Manual of Clinical Prob-
   lems in Internal Medicine* (2nd ed). Boston: Little,
   Brown, 1978, p 3.

2-M. Complications of Cardiopulmonary Resuscitation

Cerebral
   Hypoxic encephalopathy
Oronasopharyngeal
   Laceration
   Fractured teeth
   Epistaxis
Neck
   Spinal cord injury
   Vascular injury and hematoma
Lung and chest wall
   Pneumothorax and pneumomediastinum
   Subcutaneous emphysema
   Rib and sternal fractures
   Hemothorax
   Atelectasis
      Malpositioned endotracheal tube

    Foreign body
    Secretions
  Aspiration
Heart and pericardium
  Hemopericardium and cardiac tamponade
  Lacerated heart or coronary vessels
  Ruptured ventricle
Visceral injury
  Acute gastric dilatation
  Gastroesophageal, liver, or splenic laceration
Acute renal failure
Fat embolism
Volume overload
Metabolic alkalosis
  Sodium bicarbonate administration
  Posthypercapnic
Bacteremia

Reference
1. Lown B: Cardiovascular Collapse and Sudden Cardiac Death. In general reference 8, p 778.

2-N. Valvular Disease*

Aortic Valve
Stenosis
  Valvular
    Congenital
    Rheumatic
    Calcific (senile)
    Atherosclerotic
    Rheumatoid
    Ochronosis
  Supravalvular
  Subvalvular
Regurgitation
  Congenital
    Bicuspid aortic valve
      Isolated

*See also 2-F.

Associated with:
  Coarctation
  Ventricular septal defect
  Patent ductus arteriosus
Tricuspid aortic valve
  Isolated
  Associated with:
    Ventricular septal defect
    Valvular aortic stenosis
    Supravalvular aortic stenosis
    Subvalvular aortic stenosis
    Congenital aneurysm of sinus of Valsalva
    Cusp fenestrations
Quadricuspid aortic valve
Acquired
  Valvular
    Rheumatic heart disease
    Bacterial endocarditis
    Calcific aortic valve disease
    Atherosclerosis
    Traumatic valve rupture
    Postaortic valve surgery
      Postvalvulotomy
      Leakage around prosthesis
      Endocarditis
    Miscellaneous
      Ankylosing spondylitis
      Reiter's syndrome
      Rheumatoid arthritis
      Systemic lupus erythematosus
      Scleroderma
      Myxomatous degeneration
      Pseudoxanthoma elasticum
      Mucopolysaccharidoses
      Osteogenesis imperfecta
      Cusp fenestrations
      Methysergide
  Aortic dilatation or distortion
    Senile dilatation
    Aortic dissection
    Cystic medial necrosis with or without Marfan's
      syndrome
    Takayasu's disease
    Relapsing polychondritis
    Syphilis
    Ankylosing spondylitis
    Psoriatic arthritis
    Ulcerative colitis with arthritis

Reiter's syndrome
Giant-cell arteritis
Ehlers-Danlos syndrome
Hypertension
Cogan's syndrome

Mitral Valve
Stenosis
 Congenital
 Rheumatic
 Carcinoid syndrome
 Marantic endocarditis
Regurgitation
 Congenital
  Isolated mitral regurgitation
  Idiopathic hypertrophic subaortic stenosis (IHSS)
  Connective-tissue disorders
   Ehlers-Danlos syndrome
   Hurler's syndrome
   Marfan's syndrome
   Pseudoxanthoma elasticum
   Osteogenesis imperfecta
  Atrioventricular cushion defect
  Parachute mitral valve complex
  Hypoplastic left heart syndrome
  Anomalous left coronary artery from pulmonary artery
  Congenital mitral stenosis
  Corrected transposition of great vessels with or without Ebstein's malformation
  Supravalvular ring of left atrium
 Acquired
  Rheumatic
  Mitral valve prolapse syndrome
  Papillary muscle dysfunction (e.g., following myocardial infarction)
  Ruptured or abnormal chordae tendineae (e.g., idiopathic)
  Bacterial endocarditis
  Calcified mitral annulus
  Left ventricular dilatation or aneurysm
  Aortic valve disease
  Prosthetic valve disruption
  Trauma
  Post–cardiac surgery
  Rheumatoid arthritis
  Ankylosing spondylitis
  Systemic lupus erythematosus
  Left atrial myxoma

Carcinoid syndrome
Endocardial fibroelastosis
Giant left atrium

Pulmonic Valve
Stenosis
   Congenital
      Valvular stenosis
      Valvular dysplasia (e.g., Noonan's syndrome)
      Tetralogy of Fallot
      Supravalvular aortic stenosis syndrome
   Acquired
      Intrinsic valvular lesions
         Rheumatic disease
         Carcinoid syndrome
         Endocarditis
         Primary neoplasm
      Extrinsic lesions
         Neoplasm
         Aortic or septal aneurysm
         Sinus of Valsalva aneurysm
Regurgitation
   Congenital
      Absent pulmonic valve
      Isolated pulmonic regurgitation
      Associated with:
         Tetralogy of Fallot
         Ventricular septal defect
         Pulmonic valvular stenosis
         Idiopathic dilatation of pulmonic valve
   Acquired
      Valve ring dilatation secondary to pulmonary hypertension of any cause (see 2-G, "Right Heart Failure")
      Pulmonary artery dilatation, idiopathic
      Bacterial endocarditis
      Post–pulmonic valve surgery
      Rheumatic disease
      Trauma
      Syphilis
      Carcinoid syndrome

Tricuspid Valve
Stenosis
   Rheumatic heart disease
   Carcinoid syndrome
   Fibroelastosis
   Endomyocardial fibrosis

Regurgitation
  Right ventricular dilatation of any cause (e.g., mitral
      stenosis)
  Pulmonary hypertension (see 2-G, "Right Heart Fail-
      ure")
  Rheumatic heart disease
  Right ventricular papillary muscle dysfunction
  Myxomatous valve and chordae (usually in association
      with mitral valve prolapse with or without atrial
      septal defect)
  Trauma
  Bacterial endocarditis
  Carcinoid syndrome
  Ebstein's anomaly
  Common atrioventricular canal
  Ventricular septal aneurysm
  Right atrial myxoma
  Constrictive pericarditis
  Thyrotoxicosis
  Isolated lesion
  Following surgical excision

References

1. Braunwald E: Valvular Heart Disease. In general reference 8, p 1095.
2. Braunwald E: Valvular Heart Disease. In general reference 1, p 1096.

2-O. Arrhythmias

Premature Beats*
Extrasystole
  Sinus (rare)
  Atrial
  Atrioventricular junctional
  Ventricular
Parasystole
Capture beat
Reciprocal beat
Better atrioventricular conduction (e.g., 3:2), interrupting
    poorer (e.g., 2:1)
Supernormal conduction during advanced atrioventricu-
    lar block
Rhythm resumption after inapparent bigeminy

Bradycardia (< 60 beats/min)†
Sinus bradycardia
Sinoatrial block (second and third degree)
Nonconducted atrial bigeminy
Atrioventricular block (second and third degree)
Supraventricular tachyarrhythmias with high-grade atrio-
    ventricular block (rare)
Escape rhythms (resulting from bradycardia of any cause)
  Atrioventricular junctional
  Idioventricular

*Modified from Marriott HJL: *Practical Electrocardiography* (6th
ed). Baltimore, Md.: Williams & Wilkins, 1977, p 91. Copyright ©
1977 by The Williams & Wilkins Co., Baltimore.
†Ibid., p 93.

Tachycardia (Ventricular Rate > 100 Beats/Min)

	Rate		Carotid Sinus Massage
	Atrial	Ventricular	
	Normal QRS (< 0.10 sec)		
Regular Rhythm			
Sinus tachycardia	100–160	100–160	Gradual slowing with return to previous rate
Paroxysmal supraventricular tachycardia‡	140–250	140–250	No effect or abrupt termination
Paroxysmal atrial tachycardia with block	140–250	Variable (usually < 170)	May abruptly and transiently decrease ventricular rate; generally contraindicated
Atrial flutter	250–350	Variable (usually 120–175)	Transient slowing of ventricular rate, revealing flutter waves
Paroxysmal atrioventricular junctional tachycardia	140–250	140–250	No effect or abrupt termination
Nonparoxysmal atrioventricular junctional tachycardia	Depends on atrial mechanism	65–130	No effect or gradual slowing with return to previous rate; generally contraindicated

Tachycardia (Ventricular Rate > 100 Beats/Min) (Continued)

	Rate		Carotid Sinus Massage
	Atrial	Ventricular	
		Normal QRS (< 0.10 sec)	
Irregular Rhythm			
Atrial fibrillation‡	350–600	Variable	Transient decrease in ventricular rate
Paroxysmal atrial tachycardia with variable block	140–250	Variable	May abruptly and transiently decrease ventricular rate; generally contraindicated
Atrial flutter with variable block	250–350	Variable	Transient slowing of ventricular rate, revealing flutter waves
Multifocal atrial tachycardia	100–200	100–200	No effect or gradual slowing
		Abnormal QRS (> 0.10 sec)	
Regular Rhythm			
Sinus tachycardia with preexisting bundle-branch block or preex- citation	100–160	100–160	Gradual slowing with return to previous rate

Paroxysmal supraventricular tachycardia with aberrant conduction, preexisting bundle-branch block, or preexcitation (rare)	140–250	140–250	No effect or abrupt termination
Paroxysmal supraventricular tachycardia with block, with aberrant conduction or preexisting bundle-branch block	140–250	Variable (usually < 170)	May abruptly and transiently decrease ventricular rate; generally contraindicated
Atrial flutter with aberrant conduction or preexisting bundle-branch block	250–350	Variable (usually 120–175)	Transient slowing of ventricular rate, revealing flutter waves
Atrioventricular junctional tachycardias with aberrant conduction or preexisting bundle-branch block Paroxysmal	140–250		No effect or abrupt termination

Tachycardia (Ventricular Rate > 100 Beats/Min) (Continued)

	Rate		Carotid Sinus Massage
	Atrial	Ventricular	
		Abnormal QRS (> 0.10 sec)	
Nonparoxysmal	Depends on atrial mechanism	65–130	No effect or gradual slowing with return to previous rate; generally contraindicated
Ventricular tachycardia	Equal to or less than ventricular rate	150–250 (may be slightly irregular)	Atrial rate may slow; no effect on ventricular rate
Irregular Rhythm			
Atrial fibrillation with aberrant conduction or preexisting bundle-branch block	350–600	Variable	Transient decrease in ventricular rate
Paroxysmal supraventricular tachycardia, with variable block, with aberrant conduction or preexisting bundle-branch block	140–250	Variable	May abruptly and transiently decrease ventricular rate; generally contraindicated

| Atrial flutter with variable block, with aberrant conduction or preexisting bundle–branch block | 250–350 | Variable | Transient slowing of ventricular rate, revealing flutter waves |

‡Arrhythmias most commonly associated with preexcitation (Wolff-Parkinson-White syndrome).

References
1. Marriott HJL: *Practical Electrocardiography* (6th ed). Baltimore. Md.: Williams & Wilkins, 1977.
2. Friedman HH: *Diagnostic Electrocardiography and Vectorcardiography* (2nd ed). New York: McGraw-Hill, 1977.

2-P. Electrocardiographic Abnormalities

QRS Interval, Prolonged
Bundle-branch blocks
Nonspecific intraventricular conduction delay
Aberrant ventricular conduction
Ectopic ventricular rhythm (e.g., ventricular parasystole)
Drug effect (e.g., quinidine or procainamide)
Electrolyte abnormalities (hyperkalemia, hypokalemia,
    hypercalcemia, hypomagnesemia)
Preexcitation (Wolff-Parkinson-White syndrome)
Left ventricular enlargement
Periinfarction block
Hypothermia

ST Segment Changes
Elevation
  Normal variant (e.g., "early repolarization")
  Myocardial infarction
  Ventricular aneurysm
  Reciprocal changes
  Pericarditis
  Hyperkalemia (rarely)
  Bundle-branch block
  Pulmonary thromboembolism
  Myocarditis
Depression
  Nonspecific abnormality
  Digitalis effect
  Other drugs (e.g., tricyclic antidepressants)
  Bundle-branch block
  Left or right ventricular strain
  Electrolyte abnormalities (hyperkalemia or
    hypokalemia)
  Subendocardial ischemia or infarction
  Mitral valve prolapse
  Tachycardia
  Myocarditis
  Reciprocal changes
  Cerebral or subarachnoid injury
  Pancreatitis
  Pulmonary thromboembolism

QT Interval
Prolonged
  Electrolyte abnormalities (hypocalcemia, hypermag-
    nesemia, hypokalemia ["QU" prolongation])

Left ventricular enlargement
Myocardial infarction
Myocarditis and acute rheumatic fever
Diffuse myocardial disease
Cerebral or subarachnoid injury
Drugs (e.g., quinidine, procainamide, phenothiazines)
Hypothermia
Heritable anomaly
Alkalosis
Shortened
Electrolyte abnormalities (hypercalcemia, hyperkalemia)
Digitalis

T-Wave Changes

Peaking
Normal
Nonspecific abnormality
Electrolyte abnormalities (hyperkalemia, hypocalcemia, hypomagnesemia)
Acute myocardial ischemia or infarction
Reciprocal effect in strictly posterior myocardial infarction
Left ventricular enlargement
Anemia
Inversion
Normal
Juvenile T-wave pattern
Nonspecific abnormality
Myocardial ischemia or infarction
Myocarditis
Pericarditis
Ventricular strain
Acute or chronic cor pulmonale
Cerebral or subarachnoid injury
Drugs (e.g., quinidine)
Electrolyte abnormalities (hypokalemia, hypocalcemia, hypomagnesemia)
Complete atrioventricular block
Vagotomy

Q Waves, Abnormal

Myocardial infarction
Dextrocardia or dextroversion
Reversal of right and left arm leads (lead I)
Ventricular enlargement
Acute and chronic cor pulmonale
Preexcitation

Cardiomyopathy and myocarditis (e.g., hypertrophic car-
diomyopathy)
Localized destructive myocardial disease (e.g., neoplasm)
Left bundle-branch block
Normal variant (rare)
Tachycardia (transitory)
Critical illness

References

1. Friedman HH: *Diagnostic Electrocardiography and
   Vectorcardiography* (2nd ed). New York: McGraw-Hill,
   1977.
2. Marriott HJL: *Practical Electrocardiography* (6th ed).
   Baltimore, Md.: Williams & Wilkins, 1977.

2-Q. Cardiac Risk Index for Noncardiac Surgical Procedures

Computation of the Cardiac Risk Index

Criteria*	"Points"
1. History	
a. Age > 70 yr	5
b. MI in previous 6 mo	10
2. Physical examination	
a. S_3 gallop or JVD	11
b. Important VAS	3
3. Electrocardiogram	
a. Rhythm other than sinus or PACs on last preoperative ECG	7
b. > 5 PVCs/min documented at any time before operation	7
4. General status: PO_2 < 60 or PCO_2 > 50 mmHg, K < 3.0 or HCO_3 < 20 mEq/L, BUN > 50 or Cr > 3.0 mg/dl, abnormal SGOT, signs of chronic liver disease, or patient bedridden from noncardiac causes	3

Computation of the Cardiac Risk Index (Continued)

Criteria*	"Points"
5. Operation	
a. Intraperitoneal, intrathoracic, or aortic	3
b. Emergency	4
Total possible:	53

Source: Adapted from Goldman L, Caldera DL, Nussbaum SR, et al: Multifactorial Index of Cardiac Risk in Non-cardiac Surgical Procedures. *N Engl J Med* 297:848, 1977. By permission of the *New England Journal of Medicine.*

*MI denotes myocardial infarction; JVD, jugular vein distention; VAS, valvular aortic stenosis; PACs, premature atrial contractions; ECG, electrocardiogram; PVCs, premature ventricular contractions; PO_2, partial pressure of oxygen; PCO_2, partial pressure of carbon dioxide; K, potassium; HCO_3, bicarbonate; BUN, blood urea nitrogen; Cr, creatinine; and SGOT, serum glutamic oxalacetic transaminase.

Cardiac Risk Index

Class	Point Total	No (or Only Minor) Complications (N = 943)	Life-Threatening Complication* (N = 39)	Cardiac Deaths (N = 19)
I (N = 537)	0–5	532 (99)†	4 (0.7)	1 (0.2)
II (N = 316)	6–12	295 (93)	16 (5)	5 (2)
III (N = 130)	13–25	112 (86)	15 (11)	3 (2)
IV (N = 18)	>26	4 (22)	4 (22)	10 (56)

Source: Goldman L, Caldera DL, Nussbaum SR, et al: Multifactorial Index of Cardiac Risk in Non-cardiac Surgical Procedures. *N Engl J Med* 297:848, 1977. Reprinted by permission of the *New England Journal of Medicine*.

*Documented intraoperative or postoperative myocardial infarction, pulmonary edema, or ventricular tachycardia without progression to cardiac death.

†Figures in parentheses denote percentages.

References

1. Wolf MA, Braunwald E: General Anesthesia and Non-cardiac Surgery in Patients with Heart Disease. In general reference 8, p 1911.

2. Goldman L, Caldera DL, Nussbaum SR, et al: Multifactorial Index of Cardiac Risk in Non-cardiac Surgical Procedures. *N Engl J Med* 297:845, 1977.

3
Drugs

3-A. Bacterial Endocarditis Prophylaxis in Adults

	Antimicrobial Regimens
A Penicillin IM/po	Aqueous crystalline penicillin G, 1,000,000 units IM, mixed with procaine penicillin G, 600,000 units, given ½ to 1 hr before procedure; then penicillin V 500 mg po q6 hr × 8 doses.
B Penicillin V po*	2 gm po ½ hr before procedure; then 500 mg po q6 hr × 8 doses.
C Penicillin G and streptomycin	Regimen A plus streptomycin, 1 gm IM ½ to 1 hr before procedure; then penicillin V as in regimen A.
D Vancomycin	Vancomycin, 1 gm IV over ½ to 1 hr, given ½ to 1 hr before procedure; then erythromycin, 500 mg q6 hr × 8 doses.
E Erythromycin	1 gm po 1½ to 2 hr before procedure; then 500 mg q6 hr × 8 doses.
F Penicillin G or ampicillin, plus gentamicin or streptomycin†	Aqueous penicillin G, 2,000,000 units IM or IV, or ampicillin, 1 gm IM or IV; plus gentamicin, 1.5 mg/kg (not to exceed 80 mg) IM or IV, or streptomycin, 1 gm IM. Give initial doses ½ to 1 hr before procedure. If gentamicin is used, give additional two doses of penicillin or ampicillin and gentamicin q8 hr. If streptomycin is used, give additional two doses of penicillin or ampicillin and streptomycin q12 hr.
G Vancomycin and streptomycin	Vancomycin, 1 gm IV over ½ to 1 hr, plus streptomycin, 1 gm/kg IM, both given ½ to 1 hr before procedure. Doses may be repeated 12 hr later.
H Cephalosporins	Cephalothin or cefazolin, 1 gm IV q4 to q6 hr, starting 1 hr before procedure and continuing for 72 hr postoperatively.

Type of Surgical Procedure	Type of Predisposing Cardiac Condition	
	Most congenital,‡ rheumatic, or other acquired valvular heart disease, idiopathic hypertrophic subaortic stenosis, mitral valve prolapse syndrome, and previous endocarditis without known heart disease	Prosthetic heart valve
All dental procedures likely to result in gingival bleeding, or surgery or instrumentation of respiratory tract	A, B, C In patients allergic to penicillin: D or E	C In patients allergic to penicillin: D
Surgery or instrumentation of gastrointestinal or genitourinary tract	F In patients allergic to penicillin: G	
Cardiovascular surgery	H	

Source: Modified from Sanford JP: *Guide to Antimicrobial Therapy*. Bethesda, Md.: JP Sanford, MD, 1981; p 78. These are official American Heart Association recommendations (see reference 1). Other recommendations may be found in references 2, 3, and 4. Pediatric recommendations are in reference 1.

*In patients receiving continuous po penicillin antirheumatic fever prophylaxis, regimens E, F, or G may be superior, because of possible presence of penicillin-resistant alpha-hemolytic streptococci.

†Antibiotic dosage may need to be modified if significant renal insufficiency is present.

‡Prophylaxis not indicated in uncomplicated secundum atrial septal defect.

References

1. American Heart Association Committee Report: Prevention of Bacterial Endocarditis. *Circulation* 56:139A, 1977.
2. Weinstein L: Infective Endocarditis. In general reference 8, p 1166.
3. Pelletier LL, Petersdorf RG: Infective Endocarditis. In general reference 1, p 1112.
4. Petersdorf RG: Prophylaxis of Bacterial Endocarditis: Prudent Caution or Bacterial Overkill? *Am J Med* 65:220, 1978.

3-B. Isoniazid Prophylaxis of Tuberculous Infection*

Eligible persons are listed by priority grouping:

1. Household members and others in close contact with an infectious case
2. Positive tuberculin reactors who have chest x-ray findings characteristic of inactive tuberculous infection
3. Recent tuberculin skin-test converters (i.e., skin test induration has increased by at least 6 mm, from less than 10 mm to more than 10 mm, in less than 24 mo)
4. Positive tuberculin reactors who have any of the following conditions:
   a. Chronic corticosteroid or immunosuppressive therapy
   b. Chronic malignancy
   c. Silicosis
   d. Diabetes mellitus
   e. Postgastrectomy
5. Positive tuberculin reactors under age 35 who have never received isoniazid prophylaxis

Reference
1. American Thoracic Society, Medical Section of the American Lung Association: Preventative Therapy of Tuberculous Infection. *Am Rev Respir Dis* 110:371, 1974.

*Before isoniazid chemoprophylaxis is begun, it is essential to exclude active infection (for which single-drug therapy is inadequate).

3-C. Guidelines for Tetanus Prophylaxis

History of Tetanus Immunization (Doses)	Clean Minor Wound		All Other Wounds	
	Toxoid*	Antitoxin†	Toxoid	Antitoxin
Uncertain	Yes	No	Yes	Yes
None	Yes	No	Yes	Yes
< 3	Yes	No	Yes	Yes‡
≥ 3	No§	No	No¶	No

*Adult-type tetanus and diphtheria toxoids (Td) for patients > 6 yr old.
†Human tetanus immune globulin (TIG) is preferred given as 250 units IM.
‡Except if at least 2 doses of toxoid are given and wound is < 24 hr old.
§Unless more than 10 yr since last dose.
¶Unless more than 5 yr since last dose.

References

1. Beaty HN: Tetanus. In general reference 1, p 685.
2. Furste W: Four Keys to 100 Percent Success in Tetanus Prophylaxis. *Am J Surg* 128:616, 1974.

3-D. Venereal Disease: Current Treatment Recommendations

Diagnosis	Recommended Treatment
Gonorrhea	
Uncomplicated gonococcal infection in men and women	1. Procaine penicillin G, 4.8 million units IM divided between two sites, with probenecid, 1 gm po *or*
	2. Tetracycline, 0.5 gm po qid for 5 days (total dose 10 gm) *or*
	3. Ampicillin, 3.5 gm po, with probenecid, 1 gm po *or*
	4. Amoxicillin, 3.0 gm po, with probenecid, 1 gm po
Anorectal infection in men, or pharyngeal infection in either sex	Procaine penicillin G, 4.8 million units IM, with probenecid, 1 gm po
Treatment failures	Spectinomycin, 2.0 gm IM
Infection with penicillinase-producing *Neiss. ria gonorrhoeae*	1. Spectinomycin, 2.0 gm IM *or*
	2. Cefoxitin, 2.0 gm IM, with probenecid, 1 gm po
Gonococcal infection in pregnancy	1. Regimens 1, 3, 4 under "Uncomplicated gonococcal infection" (tetracycline (regimen 2) is *contraindicated in pregnancy)* *or*
	2. Spectinomycin, 2.0 gm IM
Acute salpingitis (pelvic inflammatory disease) Outpatients	1. Tetracycline, 0.5 gm po qid for 10 days (in penicillin-allergic patients) *or*

Diagnosis	Recommended Treatment
	2. Procaine penicillin G, 4.8 million units IM, or ampicillin, 3.5 gm po, or amoxicillin, 3.0 gm po, each with probenecid, 1 gm po, and followed by ampicillin or amoxicillin, 0.5 gm po qid for 10 days
Hospitalized patients	1. Aqueous crystalline penicillin G, 20 million units IV daily until improvement occurs, followed by ampicillin, 0.5 gm po qid, to complete 10 days of therapy *or*
	2. Tetracycline, 0.25 gm IV qid until improvement occurs, followed by 0.5 gm po qid to complete 10 days of therapy. Since optimal therapy for hospitalized patients has not been established, often other antibiotics are used.
Acute epididymitis	As in "Acute Salpingitis, Outpatients."
Disseminated gonococcal infection (arthritis-dermatitis syndrome)	1. Ampicillin, 3.5 gm po, or amoxicillin, 3.0 gm po, followed by ampicillin or amoxicillin, 0.5 gm po qid for 7 days *or*
	2. Tetracycline or erythromycin, 0.5 gm po qid for 7 days *or*
	3. Spectinomycin, 2.0 gm IM bid for 3 days *or*
	4. Aqueous crystalline penicillin G, 10 million units IV daily until improvement occurs, followed by ampicillin, 0.5 gm po qid, to complete 7 days of therapy

Nongonococcal urethritis

1. Tetracycline, 1.5 gm po, followed by 0.5 gm po qid for 7–14 days or
2. Erythromycin, 0.5 gm po qid for 7–14 days

	Non-Penicillin-Allergic	Penicillin-Allergic
Syphilis		
Primary, secondary, or early latent	Benzathine penicillin G, 2.4 million units IM (half in each hip) as single dose or Procaine penicillin G, 600,000 units IM qd for 8 days	Erythromycin or tetracycline, 0.5 gm po qid for 15 days
Late latent or latent of undetermined duration	CSF normal: Treat as primary CSF abnormal: Treat as neurosyphilis	CSF normal: Treat as primary CSF abnormal: Treat as neurosyphilis
Late neurosyphilis	Procaine penicillin G, 600,000 units IM qd for 14 days or Aqueous penicillin G, 12 to 24 million units IV qd for at least 10 days	Erythromycin or tetracycline, 0.5 gm po qid for 30 days
Late cardiovascular or benign tertiary	Benzathine penicillin G, 2.4 million units IM q wk for 3 wk	Treat as neurosyphilis

References

1. U.S. Department of Health, Education, and Welfare, Public Health Service, Center for Disease Control: Gonorrhea: Center for Disease Control Recommended Treatment Schedules, 1979. *Ann Intern Med* 90:809, 1979.
2. Syphilotherapy 1976: Position Paper for the Current USPHS Recommendations. *J Am Vener Dis Assoc* 3:98, 1976.

3-E. Common Drugs Requiring Dosage Adjustment in Renal Failure

Antibiotics
Aminoglycosides (e.g., tobramycin)
Cephalosporins
Ethambutol
5-Fluorocytosine
Metronidazole
Nalidixic acid
Nitrofurantoin
Penicillins (except cloxacillin, dicloxacillin, nafcillin, oxacillin)
Pentamidine
Quinine
Sulfamethoxazole-trimethoprim
Sulfisoxazole
Tetracyclines (avoid if possible)
Vancomycin

Analgesics
Acetaminophen
Aspirin
Phenazopyridine (Pyridium)
Propoxyphene (Darvon)
Methadone

Sedatives
Phenobarbital

Meprobamate
Glutethimide (Doriden)
Lithium carbonate

Cardiovascular Drugs
Bretylium
Procainamide
Clonidine
Guanethidine
Disopyramide (Norpace)
Hydralazine
Methyldopa
Digoxin
Digitoxin (for creatinine clearance < 10 ml/min)
Diuretics (except furosemide, metolazone)

Antineoplastic and Immunosuppressive Drugs
Methotrexate
Bleomycin
Azathioprine
Mitomycin C
Streptozotocin
Hydroxyurea
Cyclophosphamide
Mithramycin
Nitrosourea

Arthritic Drugs
Allopurinol
Colchicine
Ibuprofen (Motrin)
Phenylbutazone
Naproxen
Probenecid
Gold

Anticonvulsants
Carbamazepine (Tegretol)
Ethosuximide
Primidone

Miscellaneous Agents
Gallamine (Flaxedil)
Pancuronium
Cimetidine
Clofibrate
Propylthiouracil
Terbutaline

Diphenhydramine (Benadryl)
Hypoglycemic agents
   Insulin
   Chlorpropamide (Diabinese)
   Acetohexamide (Dymelor)
   Tolbutamide (Orinase)

Reference

1. Bennett WM, Muther RS, Parker RA, et al: Drug Therapy in Renal Failure: Dosing Guidelines for Adults. *Ann Intern Med* 93:62, 286, 1980.

3-F. Guidelines for Intravenous Aminophylline Therapy*

Loading Dose†	Dose (mg/kg)‡
No known theophylline ingestion in past 24–48 hr	5–6 mg/kg over 15–30 min
Theophylline ingested within past 48 hr	0–3 mg/kg over 15–30 min
Poor clinical response to initial loading dose and no clinical signs of toxicity, or theophylline blood level < 15 μg/ml	Additional 1–3 mg/kg over 15–30 min

Maintenance Dose (Continuous Infusion)	Dose (mg/kg/hr)§
Children > 9 yr old and adult smokers < 55 yr old	0.50–0.60
Adult nonsmokers	0.40
Severe airway obstruction	0.40
Mild-to-moderate heart failure	≤0.40
Severe heart failure	≤0.20
Pneumonia	0.20–0.40

*Serum theophylline determinations after 12 to 36 hr of continuous aminophylline infusion are useful.

Maintenance Dose (Continuous Infusion)	Dose (mg/kg/hr)§
Liver dysfunction with serum bilirubin < 1.5 mg/dl and serum albumin > 2.9 gm/dl	≤0.45
Liver dysfunction with serum bilirubin > 1.5 mg/dl and/or serum albumin < 2.9 gm/dl	≤0.20

†To achieve a serum level of 10 μg/ml from 0 μg/ml.
‡Based on ideal body weight.
§To maintain a serum concentration of 10 μg/ml.

References
1. Hendeles L, Weinberger M: Poisoning Patients with Intravenous Theophylline (editorial). *Am J Hosp Pharm* 37:49, 1980.
2. Powell JR, Vozeh S, Hopewell P, et al: Theophylline Disposition in Acutely Ill Hospitalized Patients. *Am Rev Respir Dis* 118:229, 1978.
3. Hendeles L, Weinberger M, Bighley L: Disposition of Theophylline after a Single Intravenous Infusion of Aminophylline. *Am Rev Respir Dis* 118:97, 1978.

3-G. Dopamine and Dobutamine Dosage Charts

Dopamine (Intropin)
800 mg (4 vials)/500 ml = 1.6 mg/ml

Weight		Dosage (µg/kg/min)*							
lb	kg	1.0	2.5	5.0	7.5	10.0	12.5	15.0	20.0
88	40	2	4	7	11	15	19	22	30
99	45	2	4	8	12	17	20	25	34
110	50	2	5	9	14	19	23	28	38
121	55	2	5	10	15	22	25	31	42
132	60	3	6	11	17	23	28	34	46
143	65	3	6	12	18	25	30	36	49
154	70	4	7	13	20	26	33	39	52
165	75	4	7	14	21	28	35	42	57
176	80	4	8	15	22	30	38	45	60
187	85	4	8	16	23	32	40	48	64
198	90	4	9	17	25	34	42	51	68
209	95	5	9	18	26	36	45	53	72
220	100	5	10	19	27	38	47	57	76

Source: Freitag JJ and Miller LW (Eds): *Manual of Medical Therapeutics* (23rd ed). Boston: Little, Brown, 1980, app IV, p 455.
*Flow rate in drops/min; based on a microdrip; 60 drops = 1 ml.

Dobutamine (Dobutrex)

500 mg (2 vials)/500 ml = 1.0 mg/ml

Weight		Dosage (µg/kg/min)*									
lb	kg	1.0	2.5	5.0	7.5	10.0	12.5	15.0	20.0
88	40	2	5	11	16	22	29	36	45
99	45	3	7	14	20	27	34	41	54
110	50	3	8	15	23	30	38	45	60
121	55	3	8	17	25	33	41	50	66
132	60	4	9	18	27	36	45	54	72
143	65	4	10	20	29	39	49	59	78
154	70	4	11	21	32	42	53	63	84
165	75	5	11	23	34	45	56	68	90
176	80	5	12	24	36	48	60	72	96
187	85	5	13	26	38	51	64	77	102
198	90	5	14	27	41	54	68	81	108
209	95	6	14	29	43	57	71	86	114
220	100	6	15	30	45	60	75	90	120

Source: Freitag JJ and Miller LW (Eds): *Manual of Medical Therapeutics* (23rd ed). Boston: Little, Brown, 1980, app V, p 456.

*Flow rate in drops/min; based on a microdrip; 60 drops = 1 ml.

3-H. Glucocorticoid Preparations

USP Name	Trade Name	Tablet Size (mg)	Relative Anti-inflammatory Potency	Relative Mineralocorticoid Potency	Approximate Equivalent Dose	Biologic Half-life (hr)*
Short-acting						
Hydrocortisone (cortisol)	Cortef, Solu-Cortef†	5, 10, 20	1.0	1.0	20.0	8–12
Cortisone		5, 10, 20	0.8	0.8	25.0	8–12
Intermediate-acting						
Prednisone	Deltasone, Meticorten	1, 2.5, 5, 10, 20, 50	4.0	0.8	5.0	12–36
Prednisolone	Delta-Cortef, Meticortelone	5	4.0	0.8	5.0	12–36
Methylprednisolone	Medrol, Solu-Medrol†	2, 4, 8, 16, 24, 32	5.0	0.5	4.0	12–36
Triamcinolone	Aristocort, Kenacort	1, 2, 4, 8, 16	5.0	0	4.0	12–36

Long-acting

| Dexamethasone | Decadron, Hexadrol | 0.25, 0.5, 0.75, 1.5, 4 | 25 | 0 | 0.75 | 36–72 |
| Betamethasone | Celestone | 0.6 | 25 | 0 | 0.6 | 36–72 |

Source: Modified from Fischbein LC: Arthritis and Related Disorders. In Freitag JJ and Miller LW (Eds): *Manual of Medical Therapeutics* (23rd ed). Boston: Little, Brown, 1980, p 388.

*Apply to only oral and intravenous routes of administration.

†Parenteral form.

References

1. Haynes RC, Murad F: Adrenocorticotrophic Hormone, Adrenocortical Steroids and Their Synthetic Analogs; Inhibitors of Adrenocortical Steroid Biosynthesis. In Gilman AG, Goodman LS, and Gilman A (Eds): *The Pharmacological Basis of Therapeutics* (6th ed). New York: Macmillan, 1980, p 1466.

2. Axelrod L: Glucocorticoid Therapy. *Medicine* 55:39, 1976.

3-I. Hypoglycemic Agents

Characteristics of Commonly Used Insulin Preparations

Classification	Insulin Preparation	Action Onset	Action Peak	Duration (hr)
Rapid-acting	Regular	IV: immediate	15–30 min	2
		IM: 5–30 min	30–60 min	2–4
		SC: 30–60 min	3–6 hr	6–10
	Semilente	SC: 30–60 min	4–6 hr	10–16
Intermediate-acting	NPH	SC: 3 hr	8–12 hr	18–24
	Lente	SC: 3 hr	8–12 hr	18–28
Slow-acting	Protamine zinc insulin (PZI)	SC: 4 hr	14–20 hr	24–36
	Ultralente	SC: 4 hr	16–18 hr	30–36

Source: Daniels JS, Fishman N: Diabetes Mellitus and Hyperlipidemia. In Freitag JJ and Miller LW (Eds): *Manual of Medical Therapeutics* (23rd ed). Boston: Little, Brown, 1980, p 355.

Oral Hypoglycemic Agents (Sulfonylureas)*

Type	Available Form (mg)	Total Daily Dose (mg)	Duration of Action (hr)	Dose Given
Tolbutamide (Orinase)	500	500–2,000	6–12	bid–tid
Chlorpropamide (Diabinese)	100, 250	100–500	Up to 60	qd–bid
Acetohexamide (Dymelor)	250, 500	250–1,500	12–24	qd–tid
Tolazamide (Tolinase)	100, 250	100–500	12–24	qd–bid

Source: Daniels JS, Fishman N: Diabetes Mellitus and Hyperlipidemia. In Freitag JJ and Miller LW (Eds): *Manual of Medical Therapeutics* (23rd ed). Boston: Little, Brown, 1980, p 361.
*Phenformin drugs have been removed from the market by the FDA.

Relationship of Plus System to Percent Glucose

Test	Percent Glucose							
	0	1/10	1/4	1/2	3/4	1	2
Clinitest, 5-drop method	Negative	Negative	Tr	+	++	+++	+++
Diastix	Negative	Tr	+	++		+++	+++
Tes-Tape	Negative	+	++	+++		+++	+++

Source: Daniels JS, Fishman N: Diabetes Mellitus and Hyperlipidemia. In Freitag JJ and Miller LW (Eds): *Manual of Medical Therapeutics* (23rd ed). Boston: Little, Brown, 1980, p 352.

Factors Causing Increased Insulin Requirements

Weight gain or increased carbohydrate ingestion
Intravenous carbohydrate infusion (e.g., hyperalimentation)
Pubertal growth
Nonuse or incorrect use of insulin
Infection
Ketoacidosis
Other acute stress (e.g., myocardial infarction, pancreatitis)
Endocrinopathies
  Hyperthyroidism
  Hyperadrenocorticism
  Primary hyperparathyroidism
  Acromegaly
Decreased activity
Hypokalemia
Drugs
  Glucocorticoids
  Thyroid hormone preparations
  Diuretics
Insulin or insulin-receptor antibodies
Insulin-resistant states (e.g., lipodystrophy)

Factors Causing Decreased Insulin Requirements

Weight reduction or decreased carbohydrate ingestion
Decreased intravenous carbohydrate infusion
Increased activity
Renal insufficiency
Hypothyroidism
Hypoadrenocorticism
Decreased dosage or discontinuation of drugs (e.g., glucocorticoids, diuretics, thyroid hormone preparations)
Intercurrent processes causing hypoglycemia (see 4-K)

References

1. Daniels JS, Fishman N: Diabetes Mellitus and Hyperlipidemia. In general reference 2, p 349.
2. Williams RH, Porte D: The Pancreas. In general reference 10, p 502.

3-J. Selected Vasoactive Drugs

Drug	Common Preparations	Dosage	Comments
Dopamine (Intropin)	1 amp = 200 mg; add 2–4 amps to 250 ml 5% D/W	Initial dose: 2–4 μg/kg/min; titrate to effect	Doses > 12–14 μg/kg/min cause primarily alpha-adrenergic effects (e.g., vasoconstriction); doses < 10 μg/kg/min cause mainly beta-adrenergic effects (e.g., increased stroke volume) and increased renal blood flow
Dobutamine (Dobutrex)	1 amp = 250 mg; add 1–4 amps to 250 ml 5% D/W	Initial dose: 2–4 μg/kg/min; titrate to effect	Doses > 20 μg/kg/min may be associated with arrhythmias
Isoproterenol (Isuprel)	1 amp = 1 mg; add 1 amp to 500 ml 5% D/W	Initial dose: 2 μg/min; titrate to effect	Doses > 10 μg/min may be associated with arrhythmias
Levarterenol (Levophed)	1 amp = 8 mg; add 1–2 amps to 500 ml 5% D/W	Initial dose: 10–15 μg/min; titrate to effect	Mainly alpha-adrenergic effects (i.e., vasoconstriction) in most vascular beds

| Nitroprusside (Nipride) | 1 amp = 50 mg; add 1–2 amps to 250 ml 5% D/W | Initial dose: 0.5–5 μg/kg/min; titrate to effect | Infusion apparatus must be shielded from light; infusion pump is required; total dose > 3 mg/kg may be associated with toxicity, especially when renal insufficiency is present |

References

1. Nordlicht SM: Congestive Heart Failure. In general reference 2, p 81.
2. Miller LW: Medical Emergencies. In general reference 2, p 417.
3. Sobel BE: Cardiac and Non-Cardiac Forms of Acute Circulatory Collapse (Shock). In general reference 8, p 590.

3-K. Drug Interactions with Warfarin (Coumadin)

Increased Prothrombin Time
Alcohol*
Allopurinol
Anabolic steroids
Antibiotics
Bretylium
Chloral hydrate*
Chymotrypsin
Cholestyramine*
Cimetidine
Clofibrate
Dextran
Dextrothyroxine
Diazoxide
Diuretics*
Disulfiram
Glucagon
Guanethidine
Heparin
Hepatotoxic drugs
Hypoglycemic agents
Indomethacin
Inhalation anesthetics
Mefenamic acid
Mercaptopurine
Methotrexate
Methyldopa
Methylphenidate
Metronidazole
MAO inhibitors
Nalidixic acid
Narcotics
Oxolinic acid
Oxyphenbutazone
Phenylbutazone
Phenytoin*
Propylthiouracil
Quinidine
Quinine
Reserpine
Salicylates (> 1 gm daily)
Sulfinpyrazone
Sulfonamides
Thyroid preparations
Triclofos sodium

Tricyclic antidepressants
Trimethoprim-sulfamethoxazole
Vitamin E

Decreased Prothrombin Time
Alcohol*
Antihistamines
Barbiturates
Chloral hydrate*
Carbamazepine
Chlordiazepoxide
Cholestyramine*
Diuretics*
Ethchlorvynol
Glutethimide
Griseofulvin
Haloperidol
Insecticides
Meprobamate
Oral contraceptives
Paraldehyde
Primidone
Rifampin
Simethicone
Vitamin C

References
1. *Physicians' Desk Reference.* Oradell, N.J.: Medical Economics Co., 1980, p 869.
2. Martin EW: *Hazards of Medication* (2nd ed). Philadelphia: Lippincott, 1978, p 423.
3. Hansten PD: *Drug Interactions* (4th ed). Philadelphia: Lea & Febiger, 1979, p 33.

*Can cause increased or decreased prothrombin time.

4
Endocrine/Metabolic System

4-A. Amenorrhea

Primary
Pregnancy
Müllerian duct anomalies
   Imperforate hymen
   Absence or anomalies of vagina, cervix, uterus
Testicular feminization syndrome
Ovarian disorders
   Gonadal agenesis
   Polycystic ovaries
   Turner's syndrome
   Mosaicism
   Resistant ovary syndrome
   Disorders with ambiguous external genitalia
      Male pseudohermaphroditism
      Mixed gonadal dysgenesis
      True hermaphroditism
Congenital adrenal hyperplasia
Central nervous system disorders
   Pituitary insufficiency of any cause
   Hypothalamic lesions
Premenarchal occurrence of any disorder causing secondary amenorrhea
Severe systemic illness (e.g., cystic fibrosis)

Secondary*
Physiologic
    Pregnancy
    Postpartum state
    Menopause
Associated with normal ovarian function
    Hysterectomy
    Severe endometritis
    Intrauterine synechiae
    Traumatic curettage
Decreased ovarian secretion of estrogen, progesterone, or androgens
    Primary ovarian failure (high gonadotropins)
        Congenital (may present as secondary amenorrhea: see also "Primary" above)
        Acquired
            Premature menopause
            Surgical or irradiation castration
            Severe pelvic inflammatory disease
            Mumps oophoritis
    Secondary ovarian failure (low gonadotropins)
        Feminizing ovarian tumor
        Hypothalamic-pituitary dysfunction
            Congenital (gonadotropin deficiency)
            Acquired
                Central nervous system lesions (e.g., prolactinoma)
                Idiopathic
                Nutritional (e.g., severe obesity, malnutrition)
                Systemic disease (e.g., thyroid disorders, diabetes mellitus, nonendocrine disorders [rheumatoid arthritis, uremia])
                Drugs (e.g., phenothiazines)
                Psychogenic causes
Increased ovarian androgen secretion
    Polycystic ovary syndrome
    Masculinizing ovarian tumor
Adrenal disorders
    Adrenogenital syndrome and related disorders
    Cushing's syndrome
    Adrenal insufficiency

Reference
1. Kase NG, Speroff R: The Ovary. In general reference 9, p 579.

*Modified from Ross GT, VandeWiele RL: The Ovaries. In general reference 10, p 368.

4-B. Gynecomastia

Pseudogynecomastia
  Obesity
  Benign or malignant neoplasm
Physiologic gynecomastia
  Newborn
  Adolescence
  Aging
Deficient production or action of testosterone
  Congenital anorchia
  Klinefelter's syndrome
  Androgen resistance
    Testicular feminization syndrome
  Reifenstein's syndrome
  Defects in testosterone synthesis
  Secondary testicular failure (see 7-N) (e.g., viral orchitis)
Increased estrogen production
  Estrogen secretion
    True hermaphroditism
    Testicular tumor
    Adrenal tumor
  Increased estrogen substrate
    Adrenal disease (e.g., congenital adrenal hyperplasia)
    Liver disease
    Starvation
    Early hemodialysis
    Thyrotoxicosis
    Hyperparathyroidism
Primary hypergonadotropic states
  Trophoblastic tumors
  Nontrophoblastic tumors
    Lung
    Testis
    Stomach
    Pancreas
    Adrenal
    Liver
    Multiple myeloma
    Melanoma
Drugs
  Estrogens
  Digitalis
  Spironolactone
  Cimetidine
  Androgens

Marijuana
Heroin
Diazepam
Gonadotropins
Phenytoin
Imipramine
Phenothiazines
Reserpine
Alpha methyldopa
Amphetamines
Isoniazid
Ethionamide
Nitrosoureas
Busulfan
Vincristine
Diethylpropion
Pituitary tumors
Idiopathic

References

1. Carlson HE: Gynecomastia. *N Engl J Med* 303:795, 1980.
2. Emerson K, Wilson JD: Diseases of the Breast and of Milk Formation. In general reference 1, p 1787.

4-C. Galactorrhea

Pseudogalactorrhea
   Intramammary lesions
      Benign (e.g., fibrocystic disease, intraductal papilloma)
      Malignant neoplasm
Chest wall stimulation
   Mechanical breast manipulation or suckling
   Chest wall trauma
   Mastectomy or mammoplasty
   Burns
   Herpes zoster
   Tabes dorsalis
   Syringomyelia

Drugs
- Phenothiazines
- Reserpine
- Imipramine
- Estrogens and/or progesterones (e.g., oral contraceptives)
- Androgens
- Heroin
- Benzodiazepines
- Meprobamate
- Isoniazid
- Methyldopa

Central nervous system disorders
- Partial hypopituitarism of any cause
- Pituitary tumors
    - Prolactin-secreting (Forbes-Albright syndrome)
    - Prolactin-secreting with Cushing's disease
    - Acromegaly with or without prolactin secretion
    - Chromophobe adenoma
    - Angiosarcoma
- Craniopharyngioma
- Pinealoma
- Basilar meningitis
- Encephalitis
- Pituitary stalk transection
- Postencephalitic parkinsonism
- Pseudotumor cerebri
- Posttrauma
- Hydrocephalus
- Empty sella syndrome
- Postpneumoencephalogram
- Other destructive lesions of hypothalamus and pituitary stalk

Non-central-nervous-system neoplasms with prolactin secretion
- Bronchogenic carcinoma
- Hypernephroma
- Chorioepithelioma
- Hydatidiform mole

Other endocrinopathies
- Hypothyroidism
- Hyperthyroidism
- Addison's disease

Idiopathic*
- With menses (Chiari-Frommel syndrome)
- Postpartum (Argonz–Del Castillo syndrome)

*Some patients ultimately develop pituitary tumors.

Miscellaneous
 Uterine-ovarian lesions
 Postsurgery
 Refeeding
 Pregnancy
 Pseudocyesis

References

1. Kleinberg DL, Noel GL, Frantz AG: Galactorrhea: A Study of 235 Cases, Including 48 with Pituitary Tumors. *N Engl J Med* 296:589, 1977.
2. Besser GM, Edwards CRW: Galactorrhoea. *Br Med J* 2:280, 1972.
3. Tolis G, Somma M, van Campenhaut J, et al: Prolactin Secretion in 65 Patients with Galactorrhea. *Am J Obstet Gynecol* 118:91, 1974.

4-D. Hirsutism

Idiopathic
Familial
Postmenopausal
Drugs
 Phenytoin
 Minoxidil
 Corticosteroids
 Androgens
 Progestins
 Diazoxide
Ovarian disorders
 Polycystic ovary syndrome
 Hyperthecosis
 Stromal hyperplasia
 Hilus cell hyperplasia
 Tumors
  Primary
  Metastatic
Adrenal disorders
 Congenital adrenal hyperplasia
 Adenoma or carcinoma

Pituitary disorders
   Cushing's disease
   Acromegaly
   Hyperprolactinemia
Miscellaneous
   Ectopic ACTH syndrome
   Porphyria
   Anorexia nervosa

References
1. Givens JR: Hirsutism and Hyperandrogenism. *Adv Intern Med* 21:221, 1976.
2. Kirschner MA, Zucker IR, Jespersen D: Idiopathic Hirsutism—and Ovarian Abnormality. *N Engl J Med* 294:637, 1976.
3. Forbes AP: Hirsutism. In general reference 22, p 1266.

4-E. Hypothermia

Accidental causes
   Environmental exposure
   Cold-water immersion
Metabolic disorders
   Hypoglycemia
   Hypothyroidism
   Adrenal insufficiency
   Hypopituitarism
   Diabetic ketoacidosis
   Uremia
Drugs
   Ethanol
   Barbiturates
   Phenothiazines
   General anesthetics
Central nervous system disorders
   Wernicke's encephalopathy
   Cerebrovascular accident
   Head trauma
   Brain tumor

Spinal cord transection
Anorexia nervosa
Shapiro's syndrome
Spontaneous periodic hypothermia
Hypothalamic lesions
Dermal disorders
  Burns
  Erythroderma
Acute illnesses
  Congestive heart failure
  Sepsis
  Respiratory failure
Protein-calorie malnutrition
Iatrogenic causes
  Deep hypothermia for surgery
  Administration of cold blood or intravenous fluids
  Iced saline gastric lavage
  Peritoneal dialysis
  Hypothermic blankets
  Antipyretics

References

1. Reuler JB: Hypothermia: Pathophysiology, Clinical
   Settings, and Management. *Ann Intern Med* 89:519,
   1978.
2. Welton DE, Mattox KL, Miller RR, Petmecky FF: Treatment of Profound Hypothermia. *JAMA* 240:2291, 1978.

4-F. Weight Gain

Increased body fluid (see 2-B)
Exogenous obesity
Cushing's syndrome
Hypothyroidism
Hyperthyroidism
Hypogonadism
Insulinoma
Congenital diseases (e.g., Prader-Willi syndrome)
Hypothalamic neoplasm

Reference

1. Foster DW: Alterations in Body Weight. In general reference 1, p 213.

4-G. Weight Loss

Drugs (e.g., digoxin, aminophylline)
Depression, anxiety, psychosis
Endocrine disorders
  Diabetes mellitus
  Addison's disease
  Thyrotoxicosis
  Hypothyroidism
  Panhypopituitarism
Malnutrition
Gastrointestinal disorders
  Poor or absent teeth
  Oral disease
  Esophageal disease
    Reflux
    Esophagitis
    Stricture
    Neoplasm
    Neuromuscular dysfunction
  Acute or chronic liver disease
  Neoplasm
  Parasitic infestation
  Inflammatory bowel disease
  Malabsorption, maldigestion
Pulmonary disorders
  Chronic obstructive pulmonary disease
  Neoplasm
  Chronic pleuropulmonary suppurative disease (e.g.,
    empyema)
  Chronic granulomatous disease (e.g., tuberculosis)
  Diffuse interstitial disease
Chronic cardiac disease ("cardiac cachexia")
Hematologic disorders
  Pernicious and other anemias
  Lymphoma
  Leukemia
Renal failure
Occult infection (e.g., bacterial endocarditis, tuberculosis)
Other neoplasms

References

1. Karsh HB: Unexplained Weight Loss. In general reference 4, p 13.
2. Foster DW: Alterations in Body Weight. In general reference 1, p 213.

4-H. Adrenal Insufficiency

Secondary
Steroid-induced suppression of hypothalamic-pituitary
    axis
    Administration of exogenous steroids
    Tumor-induced steroid production
Pituitary destruction or failure

Primary
Idiopathic (autoimmune?)
    Isolated
    Associated with other endocrinopathies
Surgical removal (e.g., metastatic breast cancer)
Granulomatous infection (e.g., tuberculosis)
Adrenolytic agents (*o*, *p'*-DDD, aminoglutethimide)
Hemorrhage
    Associated with anticoagulant use
    Trauma
    Sepsis
    Idiopathic
Metastatic cancer
Enzyme inhibitors (e.g., metapyrone)
Congenital adrenal hyperplasia
Amyloidosis
Irradiation
Hemochromatosis
Sarcoidosis
Infarction
Adrenoleukodystrophy

References
1. Williams GH, Dluhy RG, Thorn GW: Diseases of the Adrenal Cortex. In general reference 1, p 1711.
2. Liddle GW: The Adrenals. In general reference 10, p 233.

4-I. Diabetes Insipidus

Nephrogenic (see 7-B)
Central
  Idiopathic
    Familial
    Sporadic
  Head and birth trauma
  Postsurgery or postirradiation
  Infection
    Basilar meningitis
    Encephalitis
    Measles
    Mumps
    Diphtheria
    Scarlet fever
    Brain abscess
    Tuberculosis
    Brucellosis
    Actinomycosis
    Syphilis
  Vascular causes
    Infarction
    Hemorrhage
    Aneurysm
    Vasculitis
  Neoplasms
    Craniopharyngioma
    Astrocytoma
    Pinealoma
    Meningioma
    Leukemia, lymphoma
    Metastatic cancer (especially breast)
  Miscellaneous
    Sickle cell disease
    Amyloidosis
    Sarcoidosis
    Histiocytosis X
    Collagen-vascular diseases
    Anorexia nervosa

References
1. Blotner H: Primary or Idiopathic Diabetes Insipidus: A System Disease. *Metabolism* 7:191, 1958.

2. Thomas WC: Diabetes Insipidus. *J Clin Endocrinol Metab* 17:565, 1957.
3. Coggins CH, Reof A: Diabetes Insipidus. *Am J Med* 42:807, 1967.

4-J. Hyperglycemia

Inadequate dietary preparation before glucose tolerance testing
Diabetes mellitus
Stress (e.g., infection, myocardial infarction)
Pancreatic insufficiency
  Chronic pancreatitis
  Pancreatectomy
  Pancreatic carcinoma
  Hemochromatosis
  Cystic fibrosis
Drugs
  Glucocorticoids
  Estrogens, including oral contraceptives
  Thiazides and loop diuretics
  Phenytoin
  Salicylates
  Nicotinic acid
  Chlorpromazine
  Diazoxide
  Growth hormone
  Indomethacin
Endocrine disorders
  Cushing's syndrome
  Hyperaldosteronism
  Pheochromocytoma
  Acromegaly
  Islet cell tumor (e.g., glucagonoma)
  Hyperparathyroidism
  Hyperthyroidism
  Renal insufficiency
  Hepatic insufficiency
  Pregnancy
  Malnutrition and starvation

References
1. Cryer PE: *Diagnostic Endocrinology* (2nd ed). New York: Oxford University Press, 1979, p 167.
2. Williams RH, Porte D: The Pancreas. In general reference 10, p 502.

4-K. Hypoglycemia

Fasting
Drugs
   Insulin (iatrogenic or factitious)
   Sulfonylureas and phenformin
   Alcohol
   Salicylates
   Propranolol
Extensive hepatic destruction
Chronic renal insufficiency
Hormone deficiencies
   Glucocorticoid
   Growth hormone
   Thyroid hormone
   Catecholamines
   Glucagon
   Combined deficiencies (panhypopituitarism)
Congenital enzyme deficiencies (e.g., glucose 6-phosphatase)
Substrate deficiencies
   Ketotic hypoglycemia of infants
   Severe malnutrition and muscle wasting
   Late pregnancy
Intrinsic hyperinsulinism
   Pancreatic beta-cell disorders
      Insulinoma
      Hyperplasia
      Nesidioblastosis
      Functional
   Immune disease with insulin antibodies

Miscellaneous
    Extrapancreatic tumors (e.g., hepatoma)
    Pregnancy
    Severe exercise
    Renal glycosuria
    Cachexia with fat depletion
    Carnitine deficiency

Nonfasting (Reactive)
Alimentary
Functional hypoglycemia
Diabetes mellitus, mild (?)
Galactosemia
Hereditary fructose intolerance
Ackee fruit ingestion

References
1. Ensinck JW, Williams RH: Disorders Causing Hypoglycemia. In general reference 10, p 627.
2. Foster DW, Rubenstein AH: Hypoglycemia, Insulinoma,
   and Other Hormone-secreting Tumors of the Pancreas.
   In general reference 1, p 1758.
3. Cryer PE: *Diagnostic Endocrinology* (2nd ed). New
   York: Oxford University Press, 1979, p 172.

4-L. Clinical and Laboratory Features of Major Hyperlipoproteinemias

Type	Lipoprotein Abnormality*	Appearance of Plasma after Overnight Refrigeration	Serum Cholesterol	Serum Triglycerides	C/T Ratio†	Xanthomas
I	Increased chylomicrons	Cream layer on top; clear below	Increased	Increased (often > 1000 mg %)	< 0.2	Eruptive
II	IIa: Increased LDL	Clear	Increased	Normal	—	
	IIb: Increased LDL, VLDL	Clear to turbid	Increased	Increased	> 1.5	Tendon, xanthelasma, planar (homozygotes)
III	Remnants	Faint cream layer on top; turbid below	Increased	Increased	1.0	Planar, tuberous, xanthelasma
IV	Increased VLDL	Turbid	Increased or normal	Increased	—	Usually none
V	Increased chylomicrons and VLDL	Cream layer on top; turbid below	Increased	Increased	0.15–0.6	Eruptive

*LDL, low-density lipoproteins; VLDL, very low-density lipoproteins.
†Cholesterol-triglyceride ratio.

Type	Premature Vascular Disease	Clinical Features	More Common Etiologies	
			Primary	Secondary
I	No	Pancreatitis, hepatosplenomegaly, early onset	Familial lipoprotein lipase deficiency	Dysgammaglobulinemias (e.g., systemic lupus erythematosus), hypothyroidism, oral contraceptives, glucocorticoids, diabetes mellitus
II	Yes	Diagnosis of primary form possible from cord blood; premature myocardial infarction common	Familial hypercholesterolemia, familial combined hyperlipemia, polygenic hypercholesterolemia	Hypothyroidism, biliary obstruction, nephrotic syndrome, dysgammaglobulinemia IIa only: glucocorticoids, hepatoma, acute intermittent porphyria
III	Yes	Patients present after age 20; severe atherosclerosis	Familial dysbetalipoproteinemia	Hypothyroidism, diabetes mellitus, dysgammaglobulinemia

| IV | Yes | Expression in adult life | Familial hypertriglyceridemia, familial combined hyperlipidemia, sporadic hypertriglyceridemia | Diabetes mellitus, hypothyroidism, alcoholism, pancreatitis, renal failure, nephrotic syndrome, glucocorticoids, dysgammaglobulinemias, oral contraceptives, stress, acromegaly |
| V | Yes | Expression in adult life, pancreatitis, hepatomegaly | Familial hypertriglyceridemia (severe form), familial lipoprotein lipase deficiency (during pregnancy) | |

References

1. Brown MS, Goldstein JL: The Hyperlipoproteinemias and Other Disorders of Lipid Metabolism. In general reference 1, p 507.
2. Havel RJ, Goldstein JL, Brown MS: Lipoproteins and Lipid Transport. In general reference 9, p 393.

4-M. Goiter (Including Nodules)

Diffuse
Euthyroid or hypothyroid
 Endemic or sporadic (e.g., secondary to iodine defi-
  ciency)
 Drug-induced
  Iodides
  Antithyroid agents
  Para-aminosalicylic acid
  Phenylbutazone
  Cobalt
  Topical resorcinol
  Lithium carbonate
  Aminoglutethimide
 Defects in hormone synthesis (dyshormonogenesis)
 Thyroiditis
  Hashimoto's disease
  Subacute
  "Silent" (atypical)
  Riedel's disease
  Purulent
Hyperthyroid
 Graves' disease
 Subacute thyroiditis
 Hashimoto's thyroiditis
 "Silent" (atypical) thyroiditis
 Ectopic thyrotropin production
 Increased pituitary thyroid-stimulating hormone (rare)
  With tumor
  Without tumor

Nodular
Solitary nodule
 Colloid cyst
 Benign adenoma (functional or nonfunctional)
 Malignant neoplasm
  Differentiated
  Undifferentiated
  Lymphoma, leukemia
  Metastatic (especially hypernephroma)
 Thyroiditis
  Hashimoto's disease
  Riedel's disease
  Subacute
 Other lesions
  Hematoma

    Granulomatous disease
    Thyroid lobulation
    Hyperplastic lobe
    Clinically inapparent multinodular goiter
    Nonthyroid adjacent mass (e.g., parathyroid
        adenoma)
Multinodular
    Toxic
    Nontoxic

References

1. Ingbar SH, Woeber KA: The Thyroid Gland. In general reference 10, p 95.
2. Robbins J, Rall JE, Gorden P: The Thyroid and Iodine Metabolism. In general reference 9, p 1325.

4-N. Hyperthyroidism (Thyrotoxicosis)

Toxic diffuse goiter (Graves' disease)
Toxic nodular goiter
    Uninodular
    Multinodular
Thyroiditis
    Subacute
    "Silent" (atypical)
    Chronic lymphocytic (Hashimoto's disease)
Ingestion of exogenous thyroid hormone (factitious)
Pituitary disease
    Thyroid-stimulating hormone (TSH) producing tumor
        (rare), with or without acromegaly
    Primary TSH hypersecretion
Toxic struma ovarii
Neoplasm producing TSH-like substance
    Choriocarcinoma
    Embryonal cell carcinoma of testis
    Hydatidiform mole
Ectopic thyroid tissue
    Sublingual
    Mediastinal

Jod-Basedow's disease (iodide-induced)
Metastatic follicular thyroid carcinoma

References
1. Robbins J, Rall JE, Gorden P: The Thyroid and Iodine Metabolism. In general reference 9, p 1325.
2. Werner SC, Ingbar SH: *The Thyroid* (4th ed). New York: Harper & Row, 1978.

4-O. Hypothyroidism

Primary
Idiopathic thyroid atrophy
Thyroiditis
   Chronic lymphocytic (Hashimoto's disease)
   Subacute (usually transient)
   Riedel's disease
   Acute pyogenic
Iatrogenic causes
   Thyroid surgery
   Local irradiation (e.g., for lymphoma)
   Drugs
      Iodine 131
      Antithyroid drugs (including iodide)
      Lithium carbonate
      Phenylbutazone
      Cobalt
      Para-aminosalicylic acid
Graves' disease
Nontoxic goiter
Environmental factors
   Iodine deficiency
   Goitrogens
Congenital causes
   Agenesis or dysgenesis
   Ectopic thyroid tissue
   End-organ thyroid-stimulating-hormone resistance
   Dyshormonogenesis

Infiltrative lesions
   Amyloidosis
   Granulomatous disease
   Lymphoma
   Metastatic neoplasm
   Cystinosis

Secondary
Pituitary disorders
Hypothalamic disorders

References
1. Cassidy CE, Eddy RC: Hypothyroidism in Patients with Goiter. *Metabolism* 19:751, 1970.
2. Watanakura C, Hodges RE, Evans TC: Myxedema: A Study of 400 Cases. *Arch Intern Med* 116:183, 1965.
3. Robbins J, Rall JE, Gorden P: The Thyroid and Iodine Metabolism. In general reference 9, p 1325.

4-P. Serum Thyroxine

Elevated
Hyperthyroidism
Estrogens (endogenous or exogenous)
   Pregnancy
   Oral contraceptives, other estrogen-containing preparations
   Estrogen-producing tumors
Acute hepatitis
Chronic liver disease
Acute intermittent porphyria
Perphenazine (Trilafon)
Genetically increased thyroxine-binding globulin (TBG)

Decreased
Hypothyroidism (primary or secondary)
Protein loss (e.g., nephrotic syndrome)
Severe systemic illness
Cushing's syndrome

Drugs
    Androgens and anabolic steroids
    Glucocorticoids (high doses)
    T_3 (triiodothyronine)
    Phenytoin
    Salicylates
    Phenylbutazone
    Anticoagulants
    o,p'-DDD
Polycythemia vera
Acromegaly
Genetically decreased TBG

References
1. Robbins J, Rall JE, Gorden P: The Thyroid and Iodine Metabolism. In general reference 9, p 1325.
2. Larsen PR: Tests of Thyroid Function. *Med Clin North Am* 59:1063, 1975.

5
Eye

5-A. Eye Pain

Foreign-Body Sensation
Foreign body on cornea or conjunctiva
Ingrown lashes, entropion
Corneal inflammation, abrasion, blebs, dystrophies

Burning Pain
Refractive error, uncorrected
Exposure to irritants (e.g., wind, cosmetics)
Conjunctivitis
Insufficient secretions (including Sjögren's syndrome)
Corneal infection, inflammation (keratitis)

Aching, Boring Pain
Uveitis
Orbital periostitis, abscess
Herpes zoster infection
Retrobulbar neuritis
Aneurysm (e.g., circle of Willis)
Orbital neoplasm (primary or metastatic)

Tenderness, Pain upon Pressure
Lid inflammation
Dacryocystitis, dacryoadenitis (inflammation of lacrimal
    sac or gland)
Corneal foreign body, abrasion, ulcer
Conjunctivitis

Scleritis, episcleritis
Iritis, iridocyclitis
Orbital cellulitis, periostitis, or abscess
Glaucoma
Sinusitis
Fever
Headache

Reference
1. General reference 12, p 159.

5-B. Red Eye

Conjunctival injection
   Conjunctivitis
Ciliary injection
   Iritis, iridocyclitis
   Acute narrow-angle glaucoma
   Corneal foreign body, abrasion, or ulceration
Subconjunctival hemorrhage (traumatic or spontaneous)

References
1. General reference 11, p 142.
2. General reference 12, p 359.

5-C. Loss or Impairment of Vision

Cornea
Corneal edema
Keratitis
   Viral infection (especially herpes)
   Congenital syphilis
   Behçet's syndrome
   Reiter's syndrome
   Stevens-Johnson syndrome
   Allergic reactions
   Drying of eyes secondary to coma
   Mucopolysaccharidoses
Corneal dystrophies
Keratoconus

Aqueous Humor
Glaucoma

Vitreous Humor
Opacification
Hemorrhage*

Uveal Tract
Inflammation (see 5-H)

Lens
Refractive errors
   Myopia, hyperopia, presbyopia, astigmatism
   Lens sclerosis
   Large changes in blood sugar (e.g., diabetes mellitus)
Opacification (cataract)
   Age
   Diabetes mellitus
   Radiation
   Drugs (e.g., steroids, chlorpromazine)
   Hypoparathyroidism
   Congenital or hereditary causes (e.g., myotonic dystrophy, Fabry's disease, congenital rubella)
Dislocation
   Marfan's syndrome
   Homocystinuria

Retina
Degeneration
   Congenital or hereditary diseases (e.g., retinitis pigmentosa, Laurence-Moon-Biedl syndrome, pseudoxanthoma elasticum)

Macular degeneration (hereditary or senile)
Paget's disease
Acromegaly
Hyperphosphatemia
Vascular lesions*
  Central vein obstruction
  Central artery occlusion
    Thrombus
    Embolus
    Spasm
    Temporal arteritis
  Carotid or basilar artery embolus or thrombosis
  Hemorrhage, especially:
    Diabetes mellitus
    Hypertension
    Severe anemia (e.g., sickle cell, massive blood loss)
    Thrombotic thrombocytopenic purpura, disseminated
      intravascular coagulation
Detachment
Retinitis or chorioretinitis
  Toxoplasmosis
  Histoplasmosis
  Sarcoidosis
  Lupus erythematosus
  Polyarteritis nodosa
  Tuberculosis
  Syphilis
  Cytomegalovirus infection
  Bacterial sepsis, endocarditis
Retinopathy (especially diabetic, hypertensive)
Tumor

Central Nervous System

Optic nerve lesion
  Optic or retrobulbar neuropathy* (see 5-E)
  Prolonged papilledema
  Optic nerve trauma
Optic chiasm lesion
  Tumor (especially pituitary tumor, meningioma, meta-
    static tumor)
  Sarcoidosis
  Aneurysm of circle of Willis
Cerebral lesion
  Calcarine tract (optic radiation)
  Parietal lobe(s)
  Temporal lobe(s)
  Occipital lobe(s)

Migraine (usually transient)
Head injury
Hysteria

References
1. General reference 12, p 159.
2. General reference 24, p 154.

*May cause sudden loss of vision.

5-D. Exophthalmos

Pseudoexophthalmos
   Unilateral ocular enlargement (e.g., trauma, myopia,
      glaucoma)*
Extraocular muscle abnormalities secondary to surgery
   or nerve injury*
Lid retraction
Enophthalmos of opposite eye (e.g., secondary to orbi-
   tal fracture)*
Congenital (genetic, racial)
Graves' disease
Orbital inflammation*
   Acute
      Cellulitis
      Abscess
      Periostitis
      Cavernous sinus thrombosis
   Chronic granulomatous ("pseudotumor")
      Sarcoidosis
      Tuberculosis
      Syphilis
Trauma*
   Orbital hemorrhage, hematoma
   Orbital fracture with air leak from sinus
Orbital tumor*
   Meningioma
   Dermoid
   Hemangioma
   Neuroblastoma

    Neurofibroma
    Optic nerve glioma
    Lymphoma
    Metastatic carcinoma
    Lacrimal gland tumor
    Rhabdomyosarcoma
Reticuloendotheliosis (especially Hand-Schüller-Christian disease)
Orbital cyst*
Orbital varices* (especially associated with trauma, arteriovenous malformation, hemangioma)
Orbital aneurysm* (e.g., of ophthalmic artery)

References
1. General reference 12.
2. Grove AS: Evaluation of Exophthalmos. *N Engl J Med* 292:1005, 1975.

*Usually unilateral.

5-E. Optic Nerve Atrophy

Ocular diseases causing retinal degeneration (e.g., retinitis pigmentosa, extensive chorioretinitis)
Optic or retrobulbar neuropathy
    Multiple sclerosis
    Infection (meningitis, encephalitis, brain abscess, local inflammation of optic nerve), especially:
    Bacterial infection (e.g., *Haemophilus influenzae*)
    Viral infection (e.g., herpes zoster, infectious mononucleosis)
    Syphilis
    Tuberculosis
    Brucellosis
    Tularemia
    Cryptococcosis
    Toxoplasmosis
    Malaria
Nutritional deprivation (especially alcoholism, pellagra, pernicious anemia)

Ischemic disease
    Arteriosclerosis
    Collagen-vascular disease (e.g., lupus erythematosus,
        temporal arteritis, Behçet's syndrome)
    Glaucoma
    Diabetes mellitus
    Sickle cell disease
    Severe anemia secondary to blood loss
Drugs, toxins
    Methanol
    Lead
    Arsenic
    Quinine
    Thallium
Sarcoidosis
Hyperthyroidism with exophthalmos
Hypothyroidism
Congenital and hereditary diseases (e.g., leukodys-
    trophies)
Prolonged papilledema
Intracranial lesions affecting visual pathways (with or
    without papilledema)
Optic nerve trauma

References
1. General reference 24, p 154.
2. General reference 11, p 305.

5-F. Papilledema*

Pseudopapilledema
    Idiopathic
    Refractive error (especially hyperopia)
Intracranial tumor, especially:
    Meningioma
    Metastatic tumor
    Hodgkin's disease
    Optic nerve tumor
    Leukemia with optic nerve infiltrates

*Optic disk swelling without visual impairment; for optic disk
swelling with visual impairment, see 5-E, "Optic or retrobulbar
neuropathy."

Infection (meningitis, encephalitis, brain abscess), especially:
  Bacterial
  Viral
  Tuberculous
  Syphilitic
  Fungal (especially cryptococcal)
Subarachnoid hemorrhage, subdural hematoma
Post–head trauma
Pseudotumor cerebri
Vascular disease (involving retinal vessels)
  Hypertensive encephalopathy
  Collagen-vascular disease (especially lupus
    erythematosus)
  Granulomatous angiitis, other arteritides
  Central retinal vein occlusion
  Cavernous sinus thrombosis
Drugs and toxins
  Vitamin A
  Lead
  Arsenic
Respiratory insufficiency with carbon dioxide retention
Hyperthyroidism
Guillain-Barré syndrome
Hematologic disorders, especially:
  Severe anemia
  Thrombotic thrombocytopenic purpura
  Leukemia
  Polycythemia vera
Hypotony (decreased intraocular pressure)
  Penetrating wounds
  Intraocular surgery
  Uveitis
Congenital malformations (especially congenital hydrocephalus, craniosynostosis, Arnold-Chiari malformation)

References
1. General reference 12, p 480.
2. Bender MB: Neuro-ophthalmology. In general reference 25, vol 1, chap 4, p 6.

5-G. Pupillary Abnormalities

Miosis
Aging
Drugs (especially pilocarpine, morphine, physostigmine)
Corneal or conjunctival irritation
Iritis
Posterior synechiae (postinflammatory)
Pontine lesions
Neurosyphilis (Argyll Robertson pupils)
Congenital absence of dilator pupillae muscle

Mydriasis
Drugs, especially:
  Atropine
  Phenylephrine
  Epinephrine
  Cocaine
Angle-closure glaucoma
Coma, especially due to:
  Alcohol intoxication
  Diabetes mellitus
  Uremia
  Postepilepsy
  Meningitis
Midbrain lesions
Ocular trauma (especially with tear of iris sphincter muscle)
Orbital or cranial trauma

Anisocoria
Local causes
  Mydriatic or miotic drugs
  Injury to iris (d)*
  Inflammation
    Keratitis (c)
    Iridocyclitis (d or c)
    Posterior synechiae (c)
  Angle-closure glaucoma (d)
  Ischemia of anterior ocular segment (e.g., resulting from internal carotid artery insufficiency) (d)
  Disease of iris (e.g., aniridia) (d)
  Unilateral blindness resulting from optic or retinal causes (d)
  Prosthetic eye
Sphincter pupillae muscle paralysis (d)
  Cerebral disease

Infection, especially:
 Syphilis
 Herpes zoster
 Encephalitis
 Botulism
 Diphtheria
 Neoplasm
 Aneurysm
 Cavernous sinus thrombosis
 Subdural, extradural hemorrhage
 Degenerative nervous system disease
Toxic polyneuritis (especially alcohol, lead, arsenic)
Diabetes mellitus
Dilator pupillae muscle paralysis (c) (see "Horner's Syndrome" below)
Others
 Tabes dorsalis (c)
 Midbrain lesion (d)
 Adie's syndrome (usually d)

Horner's Syndrome

Peripheral causes: compression of, or injury to, cervical nerve roots, ganglia, or efferent sympathetic fibers
 Trauma (surgical or accidental)
 Mediastinal tumor (especially bronchogenic carcinoma, metastatic tumor, Hodgkin's disease)
 Thyroid adenoma
 Neurofibromatosis
 Internal carotid artery aneurysm
Central nervous system causes
 Posterior inferior cerebellar artery occlusion
 Multiple sclerosis
 Syringomyelia
 Brain stem or cervical cord tumor
 Spinal cord trauma
Congenital

Reference
1. General reference 11, p 237.

*"d" indicates the affected pupil is dilated; "c" indicates affected pupil is constricted.

5-H. Uveitis

Infection (local inflammation of orbit, cornea, conjunc-
    tiva; or meningitis)
    Bacterial, especially:
        Staphylococcus aureus
        Proteus species
        Pseudomonas aeruginosa
        Bacillus subtilis
        Coliforms
        Neisseria gonorrhoeae
    Tuberculosis
    Leprosy
    Spirochetal (syphilis)
    Viral, especially:
        Herpes simplex, herpes zoster
        Cytomegalovirus
        Variola
        Vaccinia
        Mononucleosis
        Lymphogranuloma venereum
    Rickettsial (typhus)
    Fungal (especially histoplasmosis)
    Protozoan, especially:
        Toxoplasmosis
        Amebic dysentery
        Malaria
        Sleeping sickness
Hypersensitivity reaction (especially airborne allergens,
    foods, protein antigens)
Irritant or toxic gases
Trauma (especially sympathetic ophthalmia [following
    globe perforation], following lens rupture)
Collagen-vascular disease
    Systemic lupus erythematosus
    Ankylosing spondylitis
    Juvenile rheumatoid arthritis
    Reiter's syndrome
    Behçet's syndrome
    Polyarteritis nodosa
    Wegener's granulomatosis
Sarcoidosis
Diabetes mellitus
Necrosis of intraocular tumor
Idiopathic

References

1. General reference 12, p 359.
2. General reference 11, p 245.

6
Gastrointestinal and Hepatic Systems

6-A. Nausea and Vomiting*

Gastrointestinal Disorders
Obstructive vomiting
　Any cause of bowel obstruction (see 6-I)
Nonobstructive vomiting
　Gastroenteritis
　Hepatitis
　Biliary tract disease
　Pancreatitis
　Gastritis
　Peritonitis
　Peptic ulcer disease
　Postvagotomy syndrome
　Gastric carcinoma
　Inflammatory bowel disease
　Ischemic bowel disease
　Food allergy

Systemic Disorders
Acute infections (especially in children)
Metabolic disorders
　Acidosis
　Uremia
　Hypercalcemia
　Hyponatremia
Severe pain
Acute myocardial infarction

*The causes of nausea and vomiting are innumerable. This list is
not intended to include them all. The important categories of
disorders with vomiting as a major symptom are listed, and several
examples of each are given.

Congestive heart failure
Radiation sickness

Central Nervous System Disorders
Intracranial hypertension
    Trauma
    Neoplasm
    Meningitis, encephalitis
    Hydrocephalus
Vestibular or middle ear disease
    Motion sickness
    Ménière's disease
    Eighth nerve tumor
Eye disorders
    Glaucoma
    Refractive error
Migraine headache

Endocrine Disorders
Addison's disease
Hyperthyroidism
Pregnancy

Drugs and Poisons
Digitalis
Aminophylline
Colchicine
Morphine and derivatives
Ergot alkaloids
Antiarrhythmic drugs
Estrogens, oral contraceptives
Carbon monoxide
Carbon tetrachloride
Heavy metals (e.g., arsenic)

Psychogenic Causes

References
1. Wightman KJR, Jeejeebhoy KN: Assessment of Symptoms. In Boguch A (Ed): *Gastroenterology*. New York: McGraw-Hill, 1973, p 9.
2. General reference 5, p 502.

6-B. Dysphagia

Oropharyngeal Causes
Painful swallowing
  Pharyngitis
  Herpes stomatitis
  Candidal stomatitis
  Mumps
  Vincent's angina
  Abscess
    Retropharyngeal
    Peritonsillar
  Malignancy
  Acute thyroiditis
Hypertonic cricopharyngeus muscle
Pharyngeal paralysis
  Poliomyelitis
  Syringomyelia
  Cerebrovascular accident
  Amyotrophic lateral sclerosis
  Multiple sclerosis
  Glossopharyngeal neuritis
Pharyngeal muscle weakness
  Myasthenia gravis
  Myotonic dystrophy
  Restricted muscular dystrophy
    Oculopharyngeal
    Laryngeal esophageal
  Amyloidosis
  Scleroderma
  Dermatomyositis
  Plummer-Vinson syndrome
Fixation of larynx
  Oropharyngeal neoplasm
  Scarring (especially secondary to tuberculosis)
Congenital abnormalities

Esophageal Causes
Motility disorders
  Achalasia
  Scleroderma
  Diffuse spasm
Luminal narrowing
  Proximal esophagus
    Zenker's diverticulum
    Hyperostosis of cervical spine
    Stricture

Extrinsic compression
  Lymph node enlargement
  Thyroid enlargement (benign, malignant)
Middle esophagus
  Carcinoma
  Peptic esophagitis
  Cicatricial stenosis
  Traction diverticulum (>5 cm)
  Extrinsic compression
    Mediastinal disease
      Malignancy
      Tuberculosis
      Other inflammatory lesions
    Pulmonary abscess
    Empyema
    Pericardial effusion
    Vascular lesions
      Aortic aneurysm
      Anomalous right subclavian artery
Lower esophagus
  Carcinoma
  Reflux esophagitis
  Inflammatory stricture
  Contractile ring
  Benign esophageal tumor
  Epiphrenic diverticulum
  Paraesophageal hernia
  Carcinoma of gastric cardia

References
1. Roth JLA: Symptomatology (Continued). In general
   reference 13, p 71.
2. Hendrix TR: Dysphagia. In general reference 1, p 192.

6-C. Abdominal Pain

Abdominal Disorders
Intraperitoneal
  Inflammatory disorders
    Peritoneum
      Peritonitis (chemical or bacterial) (see 6-J)
    Hollow viscera
      Gastroenteritis
      Appendicitis
      Cholecystitis
      Peptic ulcer disease
      Gastritis
      Regional enteritis
      Colitis
      Diverticulitis
    Solid viscera
      Pancreatitis (see 6-K)
      Hepatitis (see 6-P)
      Abscess (especially hepatic, splenic, pancreatic)
    Pelvic viscera
      Pelvic inflammatory disease
      Tuboovarian disease
      Mittelschmerz
      Endometritis
      Endometriosis
    Mesentery
      Mesenteric lymphadenitis
  Mechanical disorders
    Hollow viscera
      Intestinal obstruction
      Biliary tract obstruction
    Solid viscera
      Acute capsular distention
        Acute splenomegaly
        Acute hepatomegaly (especially hepatitis, hepatic
          congestion)
    Pelvic viscera
      Ovarian cyst/torsion
      Ectopic pregnancy
    Mesentery
      Omental torsion
  Malignancy
    Pancreatic
    Gastric
    Hepatic
    Colonic

        Ovarian
        Uterine
     Vascular disorders
        Intraabdominal bleeding
        Ischemia
           Mesenteric artery insufficiency or thrombosis
           Infarction (especially liver, spleen)
           Omental ischemia
Extraperitoneal
    Pyelonephritis
    Ureteral obstruction (especially stones, tumor)
    Aortic aneurysm
      Rupture
      Dissection
      Expansion
    Perinephric abscess
    Psoas abscess
    Prostatitis
    Seminal vesiculitis
    Epididymitis

Extraabdominal Disorders
Thoracic
    Lung
      Pneumonia
      Pulmonary infarction
      Pneumothorax
      Empyema
    Heart
      Myocardial ischemia or infarction
      Pericarditis
      Myocarditis, endocarditis
    Esophagus
      Esophagitis
      Esophageal spasm
      Esophageal rupture
Neurologic
    Radiculitis
      Herpes zoster
      Degenerative arthritis
      Herniated vertebral disk
      Tumor
    Causalgia
    Tabes dorsalis
Hematologic
    Leukemia
    Lymphoma
    Sickle cell crisis

Abdominal wall
  Contusion
  Hematoma
Toxins
  Insect bites (especially from black widow spiders)
  Snake venom
Metabolic disorders
  Uremia
  Diabetes (especially ketoacidosis)
  Addisonian crisis
  Porphyria
  Lead colic
  Hyperlipidemia
  Hereditary angioneurotic edema
Psychiatric disorders
  Depression
  Hysteria
  Schizophrenia
  Factitious abdominal pain
Other
  Acute glaucoma

References
1. Schwartz SI, Storer EH: Manifestations of Gastrointestinal Disease. In Schwartz SI (Ed): *Principles of
   Surgery* (3rd ed). New York: McGraw-Hill, 1979, p 1039.
2. Way LW: Abdominal Pain and the Acute Abdomen. In
   general reference 15, p 394.

6-D. Characteristic Location of Abdominal Pain Associated with Various Diseases*

Diffuse
Peritonitis
Pancreatitis
Leukemia
Sickle cell crisis
Early appendicitis
Mesenteric adenitis
Mesenteric thrombosis
Gastroenteritis
Aneurysm
Colitis
Intestinal obstruction
Metabolic, toxic, bacterial causes

Right Upper Quadrant
Gallbladder and biliary tract
Hepatitis
Hepatic abscess
Hepatomegaly resulting from congestive heart failure
Peptic ulcer
Pancreatitis
Retrocecal appendicitis
Renal pain
Herpes zoster
Myocardial ischemia
Pericarditis
Pneumonia
Empyema
Pulmonary infarction

Left Upper Quadrant
Gastritis
Pancreatitis
Splenic
   Enlargement, rupture
   Infarction, aneurysm
Renal pain
Herpes zoster

*From Schwartz SI, Storer EH: Manifestations of Gastrointestinal Disease. In Schwartz SI (Ed): *Principles of Surgery* (3rd ed). New York: McGraw-Hill, 1979, p 1044. Copyright © 1979 by McGraw-Hill Book Company. Used with permission of McGraw-Hill Book Company.

Myocardial ischemia
Pneumonia
Empyema
Pulmonary infarction

Right Lower Quadrant
Appendicitis
Intestinal obstruction
Regional enteritis
Diverticulitis
Cholecystitis
Perforated ulcer
Leaking aortic aneurysm
Abdominal wall hematoma
Ectopic pregnancy
Ovarian cyst or torsion
Salpingitis
Mittelschmerz
Endometriosis
Ureteral calculi
Renal pain
Seminal vesiculitis
Psoas abscess

Left Lower Quadrant
Diverticulitis
Intestinal obstruction
Appendicitis
Leaking aortic aneurysm
Abdominal wall hematoma
Ectopic pregnancy
Mittelschmerz
Ovarian cyst or torsion
Salpingitis
Endometriosis
Ureteral calculi
Renal pain
Seminal vesiculitis
Psoas abscess

6-E. Constipation

Simple constipation
  Low-residue diet
  Laxative and/or enema abuse
  Muscular weakness
Irritable-bowel syndrome
Gastrointestinal disorders
  Colonic
    Partial bowel obstruction
      Neoplasm (benign, malignant)
      Fecal impaction
      Diverticulitis
      Hernia
      Adhesions
      Strictures
      Volvulus
      Intussusception
      Colonic spasm
    Extrinsic compression
      Pregnancy
      Large abdominal or pelvic tumor
      Ascites
  Anorectal
    Proctitis (especially ulcerative)
    Hemorrhoids
    Fissures and fistulas
    Perineal abscess
    Rectal prolapse
    Stenosis
      Neoplastic
      Inflammatory (especially lymphogranuloma
        venereum)
      Postsurgical
    Puborectalis syndrome
  Gastric
    Peptic ulcer disease (resulting from diet?)
    Gastric outlet obstruction
    Impaired gastric emptying
Neurogenic disorders
  Decreased gastrointestinal motility
    Anticholinergic drugs
    Spinal cord disorders (especially trauma, multiple
      sclerosis, cauda equina tumor)
    Diabetic autonomic neuropathy
    Muscular abnormality
      Scleroderma

        Myotonic dystrophy
        Dermatomyositis
      Megacolon
        Idiopathic
        Hirschsprung's disease
        Chagas' disease
      Colonic pseudoobstruction
    Neurologic and psychiatric disorders
      Psychotic depression
      Senility
      Cerebrovascular accidents
      Parkinson's disease
      Central nervous system tumor
Endocrine and metabolic disorders
    Hypothyroidism
    Hyperparathyroidism
    Other hypercalcemic states
    Hypokalemia
    Lead poisoning
    Porphyria
Drugs, especially:
    Antacids
      Calcium carbonate
      Aluminum hydroxide
    Opiates
    Anticholinergics
    Tricyclic antidepressants
    Phenothiazines
    Ferrous sulfate
    Barium sulfate
    Ion-exchange resins

References
1. Deuroede G: Constipation: Mechanism and Management. In general reference 15, p 368.
2. Bockus HL: Simple Constipation. In general reference 13, p 935.

6-F. Diarrhea

Acute
Infectious
  Viral
  Bacterial
    Invasive (especially *Shigella, Salmonella, Campylobacter*)
    Toxic (especially *Staphylococcus, Escherichia coli*, clostridia, *Vibrio* species)
  Protozoal (especially amebiasis, giardiasis)
Stress-induced
Traveler's diarrhea
Food allergy
Dietary indiscretion (especially prunes, unripe fruit, rhubarb)
Gastrointestinal disorders
  Partial bowel obstruction
  Diverticulitis
  Appendicitis
  Ischemic bowel disease
  Pseudomembranous colitis
  Initial attack of ulcerative colitis or regional enteritis
Systemic disorders
  Uremia
  Carcinoid syndrome
  Endocrine disorders
    Thyrotoxicosis
    Addisonian crisis
Poisoning
  Heavy metals (especially arsenic, cadmium, mercury)
  Mushrooms
Drugs
  Laxatives
  Broad-spectrum antibiotics
  Magnesium antacids
  Lactulose
  Colchicine
  Digitalis
  Iron
  Guanethidine
  Methyldopa
  Hydralazine
  Quinidine
Acute exacerbation of chronic diarrhea

Chronic
Infectious

Tuberculous
Fungal (especially candidiasis, actinomycosis)
Parasitic (especially amebiasis, giardiasis, stron-
    gyloidiasis)
Gastrointestinal disorders
  Stomach
    Gastrectomy
    Gastroenterostomy
    Pyloroplasty
    Gastroileac or gastrocolic fistula
  Small bowel (see 6-G, "Impaired Absorption")
  Colon and rectum
    Ulcerative colitis
    Granulomatous colitis
    Diverticulitis
    Proctitis
    Partial intestinal obstruction
    Fecal impaction
    Neoplasm
      Carcinoma
      Villous adenoma
      Abdominal lymphoma
    Ischemic bowel disease
    Radiation colitis
    Eosinophilic gastroenteritis
    Familial polyposis of the colon
    Protein-losing enteropathy
Malabsorption syndromes (see 6-G)
  Deficiency of pancreatic enzymes, bile salts, or
    disaccharidases
  Small-bowel disorders, especially:
    Mucosal abnormalities
    Infiltrative diseases
    Lymphatic obstruction
  Systemic disease with malabsorption
  Drugs
Secretory neoplastic disorders
  Carcinoid tumor
  Pancreatic islet cell tumor
    Zollinger-Ellison syndrome
    Watery diarrhea and hypokalemia syndrome
  Medullary carcinoma
  Ganglioneuroblastoma of the adrenal
  Carotid body tumor
Systemic disease
  Endocrine disorders
    Addison's disease
    Hyperthyroidism

Hypoparathyroidism
Collagen vascular disorders
  Systemic lupus erythematosus
  Scleroderma
  Polyarteritis nodosa
Others
  Uremia
  Neuropathic disorders (especially diabetes mellitus,
    amyloidosis, postvagotomy state)
  Cirrhosis
  Chronic cholecystitis
  Deficiency syndromes
    Pernicious anemia
    Pellagra
  Immunoglobulin deficiencies
Functional bowel disease ("irritable" or "spastic" colon)
Drugs (see also "Acute" above)
  Chronic opiate abuse

References

1. Haubrich WS: Diarrhea and Constipation. In general reference 13, p 918.
2. General reference 3, p 346.
3. Krejs GJ, Fordtran JS: Diarrhea. In general reference 15, p 313.

6-G. Malabsorption

Impaired Digestion

Pancreatic enzyme deficiency
  Chronic pancreatitis
  Pancreatic resection
  Pancreatic carcinoma
  Cystic fibrosis
Bile salt deficiency
  Bile duct obstruction
  Hepatocellular disease
  Ileal resection (>3 ft)
  Diffuse ileal disease (especially regional ileitis)*

Bacterial overgrowth as a result of stasis
    Surgical blind loop
    Stricture, fistula
    Regional ileitis*
    Small-bowel diverticula
    Hypomotility states
        Intestinal diabetic neuropathy*
        Scleroderma*
        Intestinal pseudoobstruction
Disaccharidase deficiency
    Lactase
    Sucrase-isomaltase
Impaired enzyme or bile salt function
    Inadequate mixing (especially postgastrectomy or post-gastrojejunostomy)
    Acid pH in small bowel (especially Zollinger-Ellison syndrome)
    Excessive dilution

Impaired Absorption
Impaired mucosal cell function
    Sprue
        Celiac
        Tropical
        Collagenous
    Inflammatory disease
        Regional ileitis*
        Infectious enteritis
            Bacterial
            Tuberculous
            Parasitic (especially *Giardia,* coccidia)
    Short-bowel syndrome
        Massive resection (especially for vascular disease, regional ileitis*)
        Jejunoileal bypass surgery
        Gastroileal anastomosis (inadvertent)
    Others
        Ischemic bowel disease
        Radiation enteritis
        Nongranulomatous ulcerative jejunitis
        Abetalipoproteinemia
        Hypogammaglobulinemia
        Chloridorrhea, congenital or acquired
Infiltrative disease
    Lymphoma
        Primary intestinal
        Extraintestinal

Amyloidosis
Eosinophilic gastroenteritis
Mastocytosis
Intestinal congestion
Congestive right heart failure
Constrictive pericarditis
Lymphatic obstruction
Intestinal lymphangiectasis
Whipple's disease
Retroperitoneal malignancy

Systemic Disease with Malabsorption
Endocrine disorders
Diabetes mellitus*
Hypoparathyroidism
Thyrotoxicosis
Adrenocortical insufficiency
Protein malnutrition
Collagen-vascular disease
Systemic lupus erythematosus
Scleroderma*
Dermatologic disorders
Dermatitis herpetiformis
Psoriasis
Food allergy
Others
Carcinoid syndrome
Dysgammaglobulinemia, heavy-chain
Genetic disorders of membrane transport (e.g.,
Hartnup's disease)

Drugs
Cholestyramine
Colchicine
Broad-spectrum antibiotics (e.g., neomycin)
Cytotoxic drugs

References
1. Greenberger NJ, Isselbacher KJ: Disorders of Absorption. In general reference 1, p 1392.
2. Gray GM: Maldigestion and Malabsorption: Clinical Manifestations and Specific Diagnosis. In general reference 15, p 272.
3. Kalser MH: Classification of Malassimilation Syndromes and Diagnosis of Malabsorption. In general reference 13, p 231.

*Causes malabsorption by more than one mechanism.

6-H. Gastrointestinal Bleeding

Upper Gastrointestinal Bleeding
Peptic ulcer disease*
   Duodenal ulcer
   Gastric ulcer
   Stress ulcer
   Esophageal-gastric junction ulcer
   Marginal/stomal ulcer
   Intestinal ulceration (e.g., associated with use of
      enteric-coated potassium chloride)
Erosive gastritis*
   Drugs, especially:
      Acetylsalicylic acid
      Phenylbutazone
      Indomethacin
      Reserpine (high doses)
   Alcohol
Varices*
   Esophageal
   Gastric
Esophagitis
   Gastroesophageal reflux (e.g., associated with hiatal
      hernia)
Mallory-Weiss syndrome
Diverticula
   Duodenum
   Jejunum
Neoplasm
   Carcinoma
   Polyp
   Leiomyoma
   Lymphoma
   Sarcoma
   Neurofibroma
   Carcinoid
   Hemangioma
Ischemic bowel disease (especially mesenteric vascular
   occlusion)
Bleeding disorders (especially anticoagulant therapy) (see
   8-Q)
Others
   Aortointestinal fistula
      Leaking aneurysm
      Aortic prosthesis

*Peptic ulcer disease (usually duodenal), gastritis, and varices account for 90% of upper gastrointestinal bleeding.

Osler-Rendu-Weber syndrome
Hematobilia
  Traumatic
  Ruptured hepatic artery aneurysm
Vasculitis (especially polyarteritis nodosa, systemic
    lupus erythematosus)
Blue nevus bleb syndrome

Lower Gastrointestinal Bleeding
Anorectal lesions
  Hemorrhoids
  Anal fissures/fistulas
  Proctitis
    Trauma
Colonic lesions
  Neoplasms
    Carcinoma
    Polyps
      Adenomatous
      Villous adenoma
      Familial colonic polyposis
      Gardener's syndrome
      Peutz-Jeghers syndrome
      Juvenile polyposis
    Others
      Leiomyoma
      Sarcoma
      Lymphoma
      Neurofibroma
      Hemangioma
  Chronic inflammatory disease
    Ulcerative colitis
    Granulomatous colitis (Crohn's disease)
Colitis
  Infectious
    Bacterial (especially *Shigella, Salmonella*, pathogenic
        Escherichia coli)
    Mycobacterial (especially tuberculosis)
    Parasitic (especially amebiasis, schistosomiasis,
        whipworm)
    Spirochetal (especially syphilis)
    Viral (melena rare)
  Ischemic (e.g., mesenteric artery occlusion)
  Pseudomembranous
  Radiation
  Toxic (especially associated with *Staphylococcus, E.
      coli, Vibrio cholerae*)

Diverticula
  Diverticulosis
  Meckel's diverticulum
Mechanical abnormalities
  Incarcerated hernia
  Volvulus
  Intussusception
  Foreign body
Systemic disease
  Bleeding disorder (see 8-Q)
  Uremia
  Amyloidosis
  Vasculitis
    Polyarteritis nodosa
    Systemic lupus erythematosus
    Henoch-Schönlein purpura
    Dermatomyositis
Others
  Aortointestinal fistula
  Arteriovenous malformation
  Osler-Rendu-Weber syndrome
  Submucosal vascular ectasia (angiodysplasia)
  Blue nevus bleb syndrome
  Pseudoxanthoma elasticum
  Ehlers-Danlos syndrome
  Whipple's disease

References

1. Law DH, Watts HD: Gastrointestinal Bleeding. In general reference 15, p 217.
2. General reference 3, p 252.
3. Isselbacher KJ, Popp JW: Hematemesis and Melena. In general reference 1, p 202.

6-I. Abdominal Distention

Mechanical Obstruction
Adhesions
   Postsurgical
   Inflammatory
   Neoplastic
   Congenital
Hernia
Intraluminal obstruction
   Neoplasm
     Benign
     Malignant
   Inflammatory disorders (especially regional enteritis,
     ulcerative colitis, diverticulitis)
   Trauma
   Foreign bodies
   Gallstones
   Parasites (especially *Ascaris*)
   Fecaliths
   Enteroliths
   Bezoars
   Food boluses
   Meconium
   Pneumatosis intestinalis
Intussusception
Volvulus
Extraluminal compression
   Abscess
   Hematoma
   Neoplasm
   Pregnancy
   Annular pancreas
   Superior mesenteric artery
Obstruction at surgical anastomosis
Congenital defect (especially Hirschsprung's disease)
Other
   Radiation stenosis
   Endometriosis

Vascular Obstruction
Mesenteric artery thrombosis or embolus
Venous thrombosis

Adynamic Ileus
Intraabdominal causes
   Peritoneal inflammation (see 6-J)

Traumatic
   Postoperative
   Penetrating
Bacterial
Chemical
   Blood
   Gastric contents (perforated ulcer)
   Bile
   Pancreatic enzymes (acute pancreatitis)
Vascular insufficiency
   Strangulation
      Intramural (distention resulting from mechanical
         ileus)
      Extramural (compression of mesenteric vessels)
   Mesenteric artery thrombosis or embolus
Extraperitoneal irritation
   Retroperitoneal hemorrhage
   Psoas abscess
   Perinephric abscess
   Pyelonephritis
   Renal colic
Extraabdominal causes
   Toxic
      Pneumonia
      Empyema
      Uremia
      Severe systemic infection
   Trauma
      Thoracic
      Retroperitoneal
      Intracranial
      Spinal
   Severe electrolyte imbalance (e.g., hypokalemia)
   Other
      Osteomyelitis of spine

Idiopathic Intestinal Pseudoobstruction

Spastic Ileus
Uremia
Heavy metal poisoning (especially lead)
Porphyria

Excessive Intraluminal Gas
Aerophagia
Increased intestinal gas production

Ascites (see 6-R)

References
1. Cohn I: Intestinal Obstruction. In general reference 13, p 481.
2. Jones RS: Intestinal Obstruction, Pseudoobstruction, and Ileus. In general reference 15, p 425.

6-J. Peritonitis

Trauma
  Penetrating wounds
  Ruptured viscus
  Surgical injury
  Instrumentation
    Sigmoidoscopy or colonoscopy
    Gastroscopy
    Abortion
    Paracentesis
Spontaneous perforation of viscus
  Peptic ulcer disease
  Appendicitis
  Gangrenous cholecystitis
  Diverticulitis
  Strangulated bowel
    Small-bowel adhesion
    Incarcerated hernia
    Volvulus
  Perforating carcinoma
  Ulcerative colitis (especially with toxic megacolon)
  Ischemic bowel
  Ingested foreign body
  Meckel's diverticulum
Ruptured visceral abscess or cyst, especially:
  Liver
  Kidney
  Spleen
  Tuboovarian

Chemical irritants
  Bile
  Blood
  Gastric juice
  Barium
  Enema or douche contents
Infection
  Bacterial
    Primary (spontaneous)
    Secondary
  Mycobacterial (primarily tuberculosis)
  Fungal (rare), especially:
    Candidiasis
    Histoplasmosis
    Cryptococcosis
    Coccidioidomycosis
  Parasitic (rare), especially:
    Schistosomiasis
    Ascariasis
    Enterobiasis
    Amebiasis
Others
  Systemic lupus erythematosus
  Eosinophilic peritonitis
  Chylous peritonitis (see 6-R, "Chylous ascites")
  Familial paroxysmal polyserositis
  Granulomatous peritonitis (e.g., starch)

References

1. Isselbacher KJ, LaMont JT: Diseases of the Peritoneum and Mesentery. In general reference 1, p 1442.
2. Rhoads JE, Rhoads JE Jr: The Peritoneum. In general reference 13, p 33.
3. Musgrave JE: Diseases of the Peritoneum, Mesentery and Omentum. In Boguch A (Ed): *Gastroenterology*. New York: McGraw-Hill, 1973, p 1051.

6-K. Pancreatitis

Biliary tract disease
  Asymptomatic gallstones
  Common duct stones
Alcoholism
Trauma
  Blunt or penetrating
  Surgical
Peptic ulcer disease (especially penetrating duodenal or
    gastric ulcer)
Neoplasm
  Head of pancreas
  Ampulla of Vater
  Metastatic
Duodenal disease
  Spasm of sphincter of Oddi
  Obstruction of sphincter of Oddi
    Fibrosis
    Edema
    Tumor
  Regional enteritis
  Periampullary diverticula
Intrapancreatic abnormalities
  Duct disorders
    Congenital
    Acquired
      Fibrosis
      Strictures
      Calculi
  Parenchymal disorders
    Fibrosis
    Pseudocyst
    Abscess
Endoscopic retrograde pancreatography
Metabolic disorders
  Hyperlipoproteinemia (types I and V)
  Hyperparathyroidism
  Other hypercalcemic states
  Hemochromatosis
Drugs
  Azathioprine
  Thiazide diuretics (especially chlorthalidone)
  Ethacrynic acid
  Tetracycline
  Salicylazosulfapyridine

Oral contraceptives
Corticosteroids*
Toxins
Methyl alcohol
Scorpion venom
Infection
Mumps
Coxsackie B infection
Viral hepatitis
Ascaris infestation
Vascular insufficiency or infarction
Hereditary pancreatitis
Other
Protein-calorie malnutrition
Pregnancy
Hypothermia
Idiopathic (about 20% of all cases)

References

1. Schmidt H, Creutzfeldt W: Etiology and Pathogenesis of Pancreatitis. In general reference 13, p 1005.
2. Gambill EE: *Pancreatitis*. St. Louis: Mosby, 1973.
3. Salt WB, Schenker S: Amylase—Its Clinical Significance: A Review of the Literature. *Medicine* 55:269, 1976.

*Controversial.

6-L. Hyperamylasemia Not Associated with Pancreatitis

Mechanism of Hyperamylasemia Known
Renal insufficiency
Salivary-type hyperamylasemia
Malignancy (especially lung)
Salivary gland lesions
Parotitis (especially mumps)
Calculi

Radiation sialoadenitis
Maxillofacial surgery
Drugs
   Oxyphenbutazone
   Phenylbutazone
Macroamylasemia

Mechanism of Hyperamylasemia Uncertain

Biliary tract disease
Intraabdominal disease
   Perforated peptic ulcer not in contact with pancreas
   Intestinal obstruction
   Ruptured ectopic pregnancy
   Afferent loop syndrome
   Mesenteric infarction
   Dissecting aortic aneurysm
   Peritonitis
   Appendicitis
Cerebral trauma
Burns
Traumatic shock
Postoperative hyperamylasemia
Diabetic ketoacidosis
Renal transplantation
Pneumonia
Acquired bisalbuminemia
Prostatic disease
Pregnancy
Drugs
   Opiates (see also 6-K, "Drugs")

Reference

1. Salt WB, Schenker S: Amylase—Its Clinical
Significance: A Review of the Literature. *Medicine*
55:269, 1976.

6-M. Amylase-Creatinine Clearance Ratio (C_{am}/C_{cr})

$$\frac{\text{Amylase clearance}^*}{\text{Creatinine clearance}}$$

$$= \frac{\dfrac{\text{urine amylase concentration (mg/dl)}}{\text{plasma amylase concentration (mg/dl)}}}{\dfrac{\text{urine creatinine concentration (mg/dl)}}{\text{plasma creatinine concentration (mg/dl)}}} \times 100\%$$

$$= \frac{\text{urine amylase conc.}}{\text{plasma amylase conc.}} \times \frac{\text{plasma creatinine conc.}}{\text{urine creatinine conc.}} \times 100\%$$

Normal:	1–4%
Pancreatitis†:	>4%
Macroamylasemia‡:	<1%

Reference

1. Salt WB, Schenker S: Amylase—Its Clinical Significance: A Review of the Literature. *Medicine* 55:269, 1976.

*This ratio is independent of the volume of the urine collection or the length of time of the collection. Thus, a spot urine is sufficient.
†Mean values for three series of patients with acute pancreatitis were 6.6%, 9.8%, and 14.5%. A value of C_{am}/C_{cr} that is greater than 4% may be seen in the presence of severe renal insufficiency, diabetic ketoacidosis, or burns in the absence of pancreatitis.
‡With hyperamylasemia and normal or low urinary amylase. This picture is also seen with salivary-type hyperamylasemia.

6-N. Hepatomegaly

Palpable Liver Without Hepatic Pathology
Normal variant
Thin or flaccid abdominal wall
Depressed right diaphragm (e.g., emphysema)
Subdiaphragmatic lesion (e.g., abscess)
Riedel's lobe

True Hepatic Enlargement
Inflammatory liver disease
    Hepatitis (see 6-P)
        Infectious
        Toxic
        Drug-induced
        Other
    Abscess
        Pyogenic
        Amebic
    Cholangitis
        Suppurative
        Sclerosing
    Pericholangitis (especially ulcerative colitis)
Common bile duct obstruction
    Gallstones
    Pancreatitis
    Carcinoma
        Bile ducts
        Head of pancreas
        Ampulla of Vater
    External compression
Cirrhosis (see 6-Q)
    Alcoholic
    Postnecrotic
    Other
Hepatic congestion
    Congestive heart failure
    Hepatic vein or inferior vena cava obstruction
        Thrombosis
        Tumor
Infiltrative disorders
    Lipid accumulation
        Fatty liver
            Alcohol
            Diabetes mellitus
            Protein malnutrition
            Obesity

Jejunoileal bypass
Parenteral hyperalimentation
Corticosteroids, Cushing's syndrome
Fatty liver of pregnancy
Massive tetracycline therapy
Toxins (e.g., carbon tetrachloride, DDT)
Reye's syndrome
Lipid storage disease (especially Gaucher's disease,
Niemann-Pick disease)
Glycogen accumulation
Glycogen storage disease
Diabetic glycogenosis
Granulomatous infiltration (especially sarcoidosis,
miliary tuberculosis, disseminated fungal diseases,
Myeloproliferative disorders
Myeloid metaplasia
Leukemia
Lymphoma
Amyloidosis
Hemochromatosis
Hurler's syndrome
Alpha-1-antitrypsin deficiency
Neoplasms
Primary
Malignant (especially hepatocellular carcinoma,
cholangiocarcinoma)
Benign (especially adenoma, hemangioma)
Metastatic, especially:
Colon
Lung
Breast
Pancreas
Cysts
Congenital
Solitary
Polycystic
Acquired (especially echinococcal)

References
1. Isselbacher KJ: Jaundice and Hepatomegaly. In general reference 1, p 205.
2. Alpers DH, Isselbacher KJ: Fatty Liver: Biochemical and Clinical Aspects. In general reference 14, p 815.
3. General reference 3, 273.

6-O. Jaundice

Primarily Unconjugated Bilirubin
Increased production
  Hemolysis, intravascular or extravascular (see 8-D)
  Hematomas
  Ineffective erythropoiesis
Decreased liver uptake
  Gilbert's syndrome
  Drugs (especially flavaspidic acid, cholecystogram
    dyes)
  Posthepatitis
  Decreased cytoplasmic binding proteins (e.g., newborn
    or premature infants)
  Portocaval shunt
  Prolonged fasting
Decreased glucuronyl transferase activity
  Crigler-Najjar syndrome
  Gilbert's syndrome
  Physiologic jaundice of newborn
  Transient familial neonatal hyperbilirubinemia
  Breast-milk jaundice

Primarily Conjugated Bilirubin
Decreased liver excretion, intrahepatic
  Familial or hereditary
    Dubin-Johnson syndrome
    Rotor syndrome
    Cholestatic jaundice of pregnancy
    Recurrent benign intrahepatic cholestasis
  Acquired
    Hepatitis (see 6-P)
    Cirrhosis (see 6-Q)
    Alcoholic liver disease
    Biliary cirrhosis, primary or secondary
    Cholangitis
    Drugs, especially:
      Chlorpromazine
      Methyltestosterone
      Oral contraceptives
      Erythromycin estolate
      Isoniazid
      Halothane
    Toxins (especially carbon tetrachloride, phosphorus)
  Others
    Hepatic malignancy, primary or metastatic
    Congestive heart failure

    Shock
    Sepsis
    Toxemia of pregnancy
    Hepatic trauma
    Sarcoidosis
    Amyloidosis
Extrahepatic biliary obstruction
  Congenital
    Bile duct atresia
    Idiopathic dilatation of common bile duct
    Cystic fibrosis
  Acquired
    Cholecystitis
    Common bile duct obstruction
      Stones
      Tumors (benign, malignant)
        Gallbladder
        Bile ducts
        Ampulla of Vater
        Pancreas
      External compression
      Strictures
        Duct
        Sphincter of Oddi
      Pancreatitis
      Sclerosing cholangitis

References

1. Lewis C, Mahoney P, Arias IM: Jaundice: Clinical and Pathophysiologic Features. In general reference 13, p 182.
2. General reference 3, 286.

6-P. Hepatitis*

Infection
Viral
  Common
    Hepatitis A, B, non-A, non-B
    Infectious mononucleosis
    Yellow fever
  Infrequent
    Adenovirus
    Coxsackie B
    Cytomegalovirus
  Congenital or neonatal infection
    Rubella
    Herpes simplex
    Cytomegalovirus
Bacterial
  Common
    Pneumococcal
    Typhoid fever
    Brucellosis
  Infrequent
    Bacteremia with *Streptococcus,* gonococcus, *Escherichia coli,* clostridia
    Tularemia
Mycobacterial
  Mycobacterium tuberculosis
  Leprosy
Spirochetal
  Syphilis (congenital, secondary, or late)
  Leptospirosis
  Relapsing fever (*Borrelia* species)
Fungal
  Disseminated
    Histoplasmosis
    Blastomycosis
    Coccidioidomycosis
    Cryptococcosis
  Actinomycosis
Protozoal (especially malaria, toxoplasmosis)
Rickettsial (especially Q fever)

---

*Acute, diffuse hepatocellular injury not primarily due to cirrhosis, hepatic congestion, biliary obstruction, or space-occupying lesions in the liver.

Toxins
Industrial toxins (especially carbon tetrachloride, yellow phosphorus, trichloroethylene)
Plant toxins
    Mushrooms (e.g., *Amanita phalloides*)
    Aflatoxin (*Aspergillus flavus*)

Drugs
Anesthetics
    Chloroform
    Halothane (Fluothane)
    Methoxyflurane (Penthrane)
    Cyclopropane
Analgesics
    Acetaminophen
    Salicylates
    Propoxyphene
Anti-inflammatory agents, nonsteroidal
    Phenylbutazone
    Indomethacin
Antibiotics
    Erythromycin estolate
    Tetracyclines
    Sulfonamides
Antituberculous drugs
    Isoniazid
    Rifampin
    Ethionamide
    Para-aminosalicylic acid
    Pyrazinamide
Antiparasitic agents
    Antimony
    Arsenic
    Hycanthone
    Quinacrine
Anticonvulsants
    Phenytoin
    Trimethadione
Antihypertensives
    Chlorothiazide
    Chlorthalidone
    Methyldopa
    Hydralazine
Antimetabolites
    6-Mercaptopurine
    Methotrexate
    Azathioprine
    Chlorambucil
    Nitrogen mustard

Hormones
    Androgens (e.g., methyltestosterone)
    Corticosteroids
    Estrogens
Oral hypoglycemics
    Chlorpropamide
    Metahexamide
Antithyroid drugs
    Methimazole
    Propylthiouracil
Psychopharmacologic agents
    Phenothiazines (especially chlorpromazine)
    Ethchlorvynol
    Imipramine
    Meprobamate
    Monoamine oxidase inhibitors
Others
    Cinchophen
    Gold salts
    Allopurinol
    Pyridium
    Oxyphenisatin

Others
Alcoholic hepatitis
Chronic active hepatitis
Granulomatous hepatitis of unknown etiology
Hepatitis associated with systemic disorders
    Hyperthermia
    Cardiac failure
    Shock
    Burns
    Hyperthyroidism

References
1. Schiff GM: Viral Diseases of the Liver Other than Infectious and Serum Hepatitis. In general reference 14, p 594.
2. Klatskin G: Toxic and Drug-Induced Hepatitis. In general reference 14, p 604.
3. Klatskin G: Hepatitis Associated with Systemic Infections. In general reference 14, p 711.

6-Q. Cirrhosis

Alcoholic
Infectious
  Viral hepatitis
  Other infection (uncommon) (especially congenital
    syphilis, brucellosis, schistosomiasis)
Idiopathic
  "Cryptogenic" cirrhosis
  Chronic active hepatitis
Biliary
  Primary
  Secondary (any chronic extrahepatic obstruction)
Chemical
  Toxins
    Carbon tetrachloride
    Dimethylnitrosamine
    Phosphorus
    Mushroom poisoning
  Drugs, especially:
    Halothane
    Methotrexate
    Monoamine oxidase inhibitors
    Oxyphenisatin
Nutritional (e.g., jejunoileal bypass surgery)
Congestive
  Severe chronic right heart failure
    Tricuspid insufficiency
    Constrictive pericarditis
    Cor pulmonale
    Mitral stenosis
  Hepatic vein obstruction
Hemochromatosis
Hepatolenticular degeneration (Wilson's disease)
Hereditary or familial disorders
  Cystic fibrosis
  Alpha-1-antitrypsin deficiency
  Galactosemia
  Glycogen storage diseases
  Tyrosinosis
  Thalassemia
  Osler-Rendu-Weber syndrome
  Abetalipoproteinemia
Others
  Granulomatous cirrhosis
  Indian childhood cirrhosis

References
1. Galambos JT: *Cirrhosis.* In Smith LH (Ed): *Major Problems in Internal Medicine.* Philadelphia: Saunders, 1979, vol 17.
2. Conn HO: Cirrhosis. In general reference 14, p 833.

6-R. Ascites*

Without Peritoneal Disease
Portal hypertension
  Cirrhosis (see 6-Q)
  Hepatic congestion
    Congestive heart failure
    Constrictive pericarditis
    Inferior vena cava obstruction
    Hepatic vein obstruction (Budd-Chiari syndrome)
  Portal vein occlusion
Hypoalbuminemia
  Nephrotic syndrome
  Protein-losing enteropathy
  Severe malnutrition
Miscellaneous
  Myxedema
  Hepatoma
  Ovarian disease
    Meigs's syndrome
    Struma ovarii
    Ovarian overstimulation syndrome
  Pancreatic ascites
  Bile ascites
  Chylous ascites
    Rupture of abdominal lymphatics
    Congenital lymphangiectasis
    Obstructed lymphatics, especially secondary to
        malignancy, tuberculosis, filariasis
    Cirrhosis

*Ninety percent of ascites is caused by cirrhosis, neoplasm, congestive heart failure, and tuberculosis.

With Peritoneal Disease
Infections
  Mycobacterial
  Bacterial, primary or secondary
  Fungal (rare), especially candidiasis, histoplasmosis,
      cryptococcosis
Parasitic (rare), especially schistosomiasis, ascariasis,
      enterobiasis
Neoplasms
  Primary mesothelioma
  Secondary carcinomatosis
Familial paroxysmal polyserositis
Pseudomyxoma peritonei
Miscellaneous
  Peritoneal vasculitides
    Systemic lupus erythematosus
    Henoch-Schönlein purpura
    Köhlmeier-Degos disease
  Eosinophilic peritonitis
  Whipple's disease
  Granulomatous peritonitis
    Foreign bodies (especially starch)
    Sarcoidosis
  Gynecologic lesions (especially endometriosis, rup-
      tured dermoid cyst)
  Peritoneal lymphangiectasis

Reference
1. Bender MD, Ockner RK: Diseases of the Peritoneum,
   Mesentery and Diaphragm. In general reference 15, p
   1947.

6-S. Ascitic Fluid Characteristics in Various Disease States*

Condition	Gross Appearance	Specific Gravity	Protein (g/100 ml)	Red Blood Cells (>10,000/mm³)	White Blood Cells (/mm³)	Other Tests
Cirrhosis	Straw-colored or bile-stained	<1.016 (95%)*	<2.5 (95%)*	1%	<250 (90%)*; predominantly endothelial	
Neoplasm	Straw-colored, hemorrhagic, mucinous, or chylous	Variable >1.016 (45%)	>2.5 (75%)	20%	>1000 (50%); variable cell types	Cytology, cell block, peritoneal biopsy
Tuberculous peritonitis	Clear, turbid, hemorrhagic, chylous	Variable, >1.016 (50%)	>2.5 (50%)	7%	>1000 (70%); usually >70% lymphocytes	Peritoneal biopsy, stain and culture for acid-fast bacilli

Pyogenic peritonitis	Turbid or purulent	If purulent >1.016	If purulent, >2.5	Unusual	Predominantly polymorphonuclear leukocytes	Gram stain, culture
Congestive heart failure	Straw-colored	Variable, <1.016 (60%)	Variable, 1.5–5.3	10%	<1000 (90%); usually mesothelial, mononuclear	
Nephrosis	Straw-colored or chylous	<1.016	<2.5 (100%)	Unusual	<250; mesothelial, mononuclear	If chylous, ether extraction or Sudan stain
Pancreatitis, pseudocyst	Turbid, hemorrhagic, or chylous	Variable, often >1.016	Variable, often >2.5	Variable, may be blood-stained	Variable	Increased amylase in ascitic fluid and serum

*Since the conditions of examining fluid and selecting patients were not identical in each series, the percentage figures (in parentheses) should be taken as an indication of the order of magnitude rather than as the precise incidence of any abnormal finding.
Source: Glickman RM, Isselbacher KJ: Abdominal Swelling and Ascites. In Isselbacher KJ et al. (Eds): *Harrison's Principles of Internal Medicine* (9th ed). New York: McGraw-Hill, 1980, p. 212. Copyright © 1980 by McGraw-Hill Book Company. Used with the permission of McGraw-Hill Book Company.

7
Genitourinary System

7-A. Hematuria

Pseudohematuria (Dyes and Pigments)
Beets
Food dyes
Phenolphthalein
Rifampin
Pyridium
Urates
Porphyrins
Myoglobin
Free hemoglobin

Renal Parenchymal Causes
Primary renal disease
   Benign recurrent hematuria
   Berger's disease (IgA nephropathy)
   Post–streptococcal glomerulonephritis
   Membranoproliferative glomerulonephritis
   Focal sclerosing glomerulonephritis
   Extracapillary proliferative glomerulonephritis
Multisystem and hereditary diseases
   Lupus erythematosus
   Goodpasture's syndrome
   Polyarteritis nodosa, other vasculitides
   Endocarditis, shunt nephritis
   Hemolytic-uremic syndrome
   Henoch-Schönlein purpura

    Malignant hypertension
    Polycystic kidney disease
    Hereditary nephritis
    Fabry's disease
    Nail-patella syndrome
Other
    Exercise
    Pyelonephritis, acute
    Nephrolithiasis
    Renal trauma
    Renal neoplasm
    Coagulopathy
    Interstitial nephritis, acute
    Sickle cell trait or disease
    Medullary sponge kidney
    Lymphomatous or leukemic infiltration
    Hydronephrosis
    Oxaluria
    Vascular anomalies, intrarenal arteriovenous fistula
    Tuberculosis, genitourinary
    Acute febrile illnesses (especially malaria, yellow fever, smallpox)
    Papillary necrosis
    Renal infarction (acute renal artery occlusion)
    Renal vein thrombosis

Lower Urinary Tract Causes

Congenital anomalies (e.g., ureterocele)
Neoplasms (bladder, ureter, prostate, urethra), benign or malignant
Cystitis, prostatitis, urethritis
Calculi
Trauma
Foreign body
Coagulopathy
Varices (renal pelvis, ureter, bladder)
Radiation cystitis
Drugs (especially cyclophosphamide, anticoagulants)
Schistosomiasis
Tuberculosis

Non–Urinary Tract Causes

Neoplasm of adjacent organs
Diverticulitis
Pelvic inflammatory disease
Appendicitis

Reference
1. Glassock RJ: Clinical Aspects of Acute, Rapidly-Progressive, and Chronic Glomerulonephritis. In general reference 18, p 691.

7-B. Polyuria

Central diabetes insipidus (see 4-I)
Renal disease
    Nephrogenic diabetes insipidus, congenital
    Chronic renal insufficiency (especially tubulointerstitial
        disease)
    Diuretic phase of acute renal failure
    Postobstructive diuresis, partial or intermittent
        obstruction
    Hypercalcemic nephropathy
    Hypokalemic nephropathy
    Sickle cell trait or disease
    Multiple myeloma
    Amyloidosis
    Sjögren's syndrome
Osmotic diuresis
    Diabetes mellitus
    Mannitol or urea administration
    Hyperalimentation
    Tube feedings
Drugs
    Alcohol
    Phenytoin
    Lithium
    Demeclocycline
    Amphotericin B
    Chlorpromazine
    Thioridazine
    Propoxyphene
    Methoxyflurane
    Colchicine
    Vinblastine

    Diuretics
    Clonidine
    Narcotic antagonists
Water load
    Psychogenic polydipsia
    Intravenous fluid therapy
    Resorption of edema fluid

References
1. Streeten DHP, Moses AM, Miller M: Disorders of the Neurohypophysis. In general reference 1, p 1684.
2. Schrier RW, Berl T: Disorders of Water Metabolism. In general reference 17, p 1.

7-C. Proteinuria

Benign/Physiologic
Fever
Exercise
Orthostatic
Contrast dye

Usually Nonnephrotic
Chronic pyelonephritis
Nephrosclerosis
Malignant hypertension
Interstitial nephritis
Acute tubular necrosis
Urinary tract obstruction
Nephrolithiasis
Renal neoplasm
Renal trauma
Polycystic kidney disease
Hereditary nephritis
Renal tubular diseases
    Fanconi syndrome
    Renal tubular acidosis
Schistosomiasis
Renal tuberculosis

Usually Nephrotic
Primary renal disease, especially:
    Lipoid nephrosis
    Membranous glomerulonephritis
    Membranoproliferative glomerulonephritis
    Focal sclerosing glomerulonephritis
    Rapidly progressive glomerulonephritis
Systemic disease
    Lupus erythematosus
    Scleroderma
    Polyarteritis nodosa
    Wegener's granulomatosis
    Goodpasture's syndrome
    Henoch-Schönlein purpura
    Mixed cryoglobulinemia
    Hemolytic-uremic syndrome
    Myxedema
    Graves' disease
    Diabetes mellitus
    Amyloidosis
    Multiple myeloma
    Sickle cell disease
    Neoplasm (especially lung, colon, stomach)
    Hodgkin's disease, other lymphomas
Toxins, drugs
    Gold
    Mercury
    Penicillamine
    Bismuth
    Antimony
    Anticonvulsants (e.g., trimethadione)
    Heroin
    Lead
    Probenecid
Allergens
    Pollens
    Poison ivy
    Snakebite
    Bee or insect stings
    Serum sickness
Infection
    Streptococcal infection
    Hepatitis B
    Syphilis
    Malaria
    Helminth infestation
    Leprosy
    Tuberculosis
    Infective endocarditis

Miscellaneous
 Congestive heart failure
 Tricuspid insufficiency
 Constrictive pericarditis
 Pregnancy (toxemia)
 Renal vein thrombosis, inferior vena cava obstruction
 Massive obesity
 Hereditary diseases, especially:
  Congenital nephrotic syndrome
  Alport's syndrome
  Fabry's disease
  Alpha-1 antitrypsin deficiency
  Nail-patella syndrome

References

1. Glassock RJ, Brenner BM: The Major Glomerulopathies. In general reference 1, p 1311.
2. Glassock RJ, Cohen AH, Bennett CM, Martinez-Maldonado M: Primary Glomerular Diseases. In general reference 16, p 1351.
3. Glassock RJ, Cohen AH: Secondary Glomerular Diseases. In general reference 16, p 1493.

7-D. Glomerulopathy

Primary Renal Disease
Lipoid nephrosis
Membranous glomerulonephritis
Membranoproliferative glomerulonephritis
Focal glomerulosclerosis
Rapidly progressive glomerulonephritis
IgA nephropathy

Infection
Bacterial, especially:
 Streptococcal
 Endocarditis
 Shunt (hydrocephalic) infection
 Septicemia, especially pneumococcal or staphylococcal
 Meningitis

Viral, especially:
    Hepatitis
    Mononucleosis
    Rubella
    Varicella
    Mumps
    Cytomegalovirus
Syphilis
Malaria
Tuberculosis
Parasitic infestation

Systemic Disease
Diabetes mellitus
Goodpasture's syndrome
Polyarteritis nodosa
Wegener's granulomatosis
Lupus erythematosus
Scleroderma
Rheumatoid arthritis
Erythema multiforme
Henoch-Schönlein purpura
Amyloidosis
Multiple myeloma
Waldenström's macroglobulinemia
Mixed cryoglobulinemia
Hodgkin's disease, other lymphoma
Solid tumors (especially lung, stomach, colon)
Hemolytic-uremic syndrome
Postpartum renal failure
Thrombotic thrombocytopenic purpura
Toxemia of pregnancy
Sickle cell disease
Hepatic cirrhosis

Drugs, Toxins
Mercury
Bismuth
Gold
Thallium
Penicillamine
Probenecid
Heroin
Amphetamines
Trimethadione
Sulfonamides

Other
Radiation
Hereditary nephritis
Fabry's disease
Nail-patella syndrome
Congenital nephrotic syndrome
Transplant rejection

References
1. Glassock RJ, Cohen AH, Bennett CM, Martinez-Maldonado M: Primary Glomerular Diseases. In general reference 16, p 1351.
2. Glassock RJ, Cohen AH: Secondary Glomerular Diseases. In general reference 16, p 1493.
3. Glassock RJ, McIntosh RM: Clinical and Immunopathological Aspects of Human Glomerular Disease. In general reference 17, p 521.

7-E. Interstitial Nephropathy

Idiopathic
Pyelonephritis, acute or chronic
Papillary necrosis
Drugs
   Analgesics
   Methicillin and penicillin analogues
   Sulfonamides
   Rifampin
   Furosemide
   Thiazides
   Allopurinol
   Phenylbutazone
   Phenytoin
   Phenindione
   Lithium
   Para-aminosalicylic acid
   Polymyxins
Heavy metals
   Lead
   Cadmium

Uranium
Copper
Beryllium
Oxalate deposition
  Hereditary
  Small-bowel disease or resection
  Ethylene glycol intoxication
  Methoxyflurane anesthesia
Uric acid deposition
  Gout
  Chemotherapy of leukemia or lymphoma
Hypercalcemia
  Hyperparathyroidism
  Neoplasm, multiple myeloma
  Milk-alkali syndrome
  Sarcoidosis
Hypokalemia
Radiation
Neoplastic infiltration (leukemia, lymphoma, multiple
  myeloma)
Vascular causes
  Nephrosclerosis
  Renal artery stenosis
  Atheroembolic disease
  Sickle cell trait or disease
Urinary tract obstruction, vesicoureteral reflux
Hereditary causes
  Hereditary nephritis
  Medullary sponge kidney
  Medullary cystic disease
  Polycystic kidney disease
  Cystinosis
  Fabry's disease
Lupus erythematosus
Sjögren's syndrome
Amyloidosis
Balkan nephropathy
Transplant rejection

Reference
1. Cotran RS: Tubulointerstitial Diseases. In general reference 16, p 1633.

7-F. Renal Tubular Acidosis

Distal (Type I)
Pyelonephritis
Obstructive uropathy
Cirrhosis of the liver
Drugs, toxins
  Amphotericin B
  Analgesics
  Toluene
  Lithium
  Cyclamate
Nephrocalcinosis, especially:
  Primary hyperparathyroidism
  Vitamin D intoxication
  Primary hypercalciuria
  Medullary sponge kidney
  Hyperthyroidism
  Fabry's disease
  Wilson's disease
Hypergammaglobulinemic states, especially:
  Hyperglobulinemic purpura
  Cryoglobulinemia
  Familial hypergammaglobulinemia
Sjögren's syndrome
Systemic lupus erythematosus
Thyroiditis
Sickle cell disease
Ehlers-Danlos syndrome
Hereditary elliptocytosis
Leprosy
Fibrosing alveolitis
Primary biliary cirrhosis
Chronic active hepatitis
Renal transplantation
Idiopathic (sporadic or hereditary)

Proximal (Type II)
Primary (sporadic or hereditary)
Transient (infants)
Carbonic anhydrase deficiency (including
  acetazolamide-induced)
Fanconi syndrome (multiple proximal tubular defects)
  Cystinosis
  Tyrosinemia
  Lowe's syndrome
  Wilson's disease

Hereditary fructose intolerance
Pyruvate carboxylase deficiency
Multiple myeloma
Amyloidosis
Vitamin D deficiency or dependency
Sjögren's syndrome
Medullary cystic disease
Outdated tetracycline
Streptozotocin
Lead
Cadmium
Mercury
Paroxysmal nocturnal hemoglobinuria
Osteopetrosis
Renal transplantation

Other
   Mineralocorticoid deficiency
   Adrenal insufficiency (see 4-H)
   Congenital enzyme defects (e.g., 21-hydroxylase deficiency)
Aldosterone deficiency
   Isolated
   Hyporeninemic hypoaldosteronism
      Diabetes mellitus
      Tubulointerstitial disease
Chronic glomerular disease

References
1. Cogan MG, Rector FC, Seldin DW: Acid-Base Disorders. In general reference 16, p 841.
2. Kaehny WD, Gabow PA: Pathogenesis and Management of Metabolic Acidosis and Alkalosis. In general reference 17, p 115.

7-G. Urinary Tract Obstruction

Urethral
Congenital urethral stenosis, web, atresia
Posterior urethral valves
Inflammation
Trauma

Bladder Neck
Prostatic hypertrophy
Carcinoma (prostate, bladder)
Bladder infection
Functional
    Neuropathy (peripheral neuropathy, spinal cord injury)
    Drugs (parasympatholytics, ganglionic blockers)

Ureteral
Ureteral-pelvic junction stricture
Intraureteral
    Clots
    Pyogenic debris
    Stones
    Crystals (especially sulfa, uric acid)
    Papillae (necrosed)
    Edema
    Tumor
Extraureteral
    Endometriosis
    Retroperitoneal tumor or metastases, especially:
        Cervix
        Endometrium
        Prostate
        Lymphoma
        Sarcoma
    Fibrosis
        Idiopathic
        Associated with inflammation, drugs (e.g., methyser-
            gide), radiation
    Surgical ligation
    Retroperitoneal hemorrhage

References
1. Brenner BM, Humes HD: Urinary Tract Obstruction. In
    general reference 1, p 1353.
2. Guggenheim SJ, Schrier RW: Obstructive Nephrop-
    athy: Pathophysiology and Management. In general
    reference 17, p 443.

7-H. Nephrolithiasis

Calcium-Containing Stones
Primary hypercalciuria (absorptive, renal-leak) and/or
     hyperuricosuria
Primary hyperparathyroidism
Renal tubular acidosis, distal
Carbonic anhydrase inhibitors (e.g., acetazolamide)
Medullary sponge kidney
Malignancy with hypercalcemia
Vitamin D excess
Sarcoidosis
Hypoparathyroidism
Immobilization
Milk-alkali syndrome
Cushing's disease or syndrome
Hyperthyroidism
Oxaluria
   Primary
   Associated with increased dietary oxalate
   Fat malabsorption
   Ileal resection
   Jejunoileal bypass
Idiopathic

Uric Acid Stones
Gout
Leukemia, lymphoma (especially after chemotherapy)
Decreased output states
Lesch-Nyhan syndrome
Ileostomy
Gastrointestinal disorders associated with chronic
     diarrhea

Cystine Stones
Cystinuria

Magnesium Ammonium Phosphate Stones (Struvite)
Chronic infection with urea-splitting organisms

Reference
1. Smith LH: Urolithiasis. In general reference 18, p 893.

7-I. Acute Renal Failure

Prerenal Azotemia
Hypovolemia
  Hemorrhage
  Gastrointestinal losses
  Burns
  Third spacing (e.g., intestinal ileus)
  Sweating
  Diuretics
Decreased effective circulating volume
  Cirrhosis/ascites, hepatorenal syndrome
  Nephrotic syndrome
  Cardiac causes (e.g., congestive heart failure, pericardial tamponade)
Catabolic states
  Starvation with stress
  Fever
  Infection
  Postsurgical state
  Steroids
  Tetracycline
Blood in gastrointestinal tract, hematoma
Hyperalimentation

Drugs, Toxins
Heavy metals
  Mercury
  Arsenic
  Uranium
  Bismuth
  Copper
  Platinum
Carbon tetrachloride, other organic solvents
Ethylene glycol
Pesticides
Fungicides
X-ray contrast media
Radiation
Antibiotics
  Penicillin
  Tetracycline
  Aminoglycosides
  Cephalosporins
  Amphotericin B
  Sulfonamides
  Rifampin
  Polymyxin

Other drugs
   Phenytoin
   Nonsteroidal anti-inflammatory agents (especially
      phenylbutazone)
   Phenindione
   Methoxyflurane
   Furosemide
   Acetaminophen
   Ethylenediaminetetraacetic acid (EDTA)

Ischemic Disorders
Major trauma, surgery
Massive hemorrhage, severe volume depletion
Pancreatitis
Septic shock
Crush injury
Hemolysis, transfusion reaction
Rhabdomyolysis

Glomerular/Vascular Disease
Poststreptococcal glomerulonephritis
Systemic lupus erythematosus
Scleroderma
Polyarteritis nodosa, hypersensitivity angiitis
Henoch-Schönlein purpura
Bacterial endocarditis
Serum sickness
Goodpasture's syndrome
Idiopathic, rapidly progressive glomerulonephritis
Wegener's granulomatosis
Drug-induced vasculitis
Malignant hypertension
Hemolytic-uremic syndrome
Thrombotic thrombocytopenic purpura
Toxemia of pregnancy
Postpartum renal failure
Transplant rejection

Interstitial/Intratubular Diseases
Interstitial nephritis (see 7-E)
   Drugs
   Oxalosis
   Idiopathic
Pyelonephritis, papillary necrosis
Hyperuricemia
Hypercalcemia

Major Vessel Disease
Renal artery thrombi, emboli, stenosis
Renal vein or inferior vena cava thrombosis
Dissecting aneurysm (aorta with or without renal arteries)

Postrenal Causes*
Urethral obstruction
Bladder neck obstruction
Ureteral obstruction

References
1. Levinsky NG, Alexander EA, Venkatachalam MA: Acute Renal Failure. In general reference 16, p 1181.
2. Schrier RW, Conger JD: Acute Renal Failure: Pathogenesis, Diagnosis, and Management. In general reference 17, p 375.

*See 7-G.

7-J. Renal Failure, Reversible Factors

Infection
Obstruction
Volume depletion
Drugs, toxins
Hypertension
Congestive heart failure
Pericardial tamponade
Hypercalcemia
Hyperuricemia
Hypokalemia

Reference
1. Alfrey AC: Chronic Renal Failure: Manifestations and Pathogenesis. In general reference 17, p 409.

7-K. Urinary Diagnostic Indices

	Prerenal Azotemia	Oliguric Acute Renal Failure
Urine osmolality, mOsm/kg H_2O	>500	<350
Urine Na^+, mEq/L	<20	>40
Urine/plasma urea nitrogen	>8	<3
Urine/plasma creatinine	>40	<20
*Fractional excretion of Na^+, %	<1	>1

Source: Modified from Miller TR, Anderson RJ, Linas SL, et al: Urinary Diagnostic Indices in Acute Renal Failure: A Prospective Study. *Ann Intern Med* 89:49, 1978. These indices are useful only in oliguric states.

*Fractional excretion of $Na^+ = \dfrac{\text{urine } Na^+}{\text{plasma } Na^+} \times \dfrac{\text{plasma creatinine}}{\text{urine creatinine}} \times 100\%$

7-L. Chronic Renal Failure

*Glomerulopathy, Primary Renal**
Excluding lipoid nephrosis

*Glomerulopathy Associated with Systemic Disease**

Genetically Transmitted Disease
Polycystic kidney disease
Hereditary nephritis
Fabry's disease
Oxalosis
Cystinosis
Medullary cystic disease

Medullary sponge kidney
Nail-patella syndrome
Congenital nephrotic syndrome

Vascular Disease
Nephrosclerosis
Malignant hypertension
Cortical necrosis
Renal artery stenosis, thrombosis, emboli
Renal vein thrombosis, inferior vena cava thrombosis

Interstitial Disease†
Drugs: analgesics only
Heavy metals: Lead, cadmium, beryllium

Urinary Tract Obstruction‡

Reference
1. General references 16, 17, and 18.

*See 7-D.
†See 7-E.
‡See 7-G.

7-M. Indications for Dialysis

Chemical Criteria
Volume overload
Serum $K^+ > 6$ mEq/L (on medical management)
Serum $HCO_3^- < 10$ mEq/L, pH < 7.20
Blood urea nitrogen > 100 to 200 mg/dl
Serum creatinine > 10 to 20 mg/dl

Symptomatic Criteria
Central nervous system symptoms (e.g., lethargy, confu-
sion, seizures, asterixis)
Gastrointestinal symptoms (e.g., nausea, vomiting)

Pericarditis
Bleeding diathesis

Miscellaneous Indications (in Absence of Renal Failure)
Hypercalcemia
Hypermagnesemia
Hyperuricemia
Hypernatremia
Hypothermia
Removal of drugs or toxins

Reference

1. Shinaberger JH: Indications for Dialysis. In Massry SG,
   Sellers AL (Eds): *Clinical Aspects of Uremia and
   Dialysis.* Springfield, Ill.: Thomas, 1976, p 490.

7-N. Impotence

Aging
Psychogenic causes
Testicular causes (primary or secondary)
   Congenital hypogonadism (especially Frohlich's syn-
      drome, Klinefelter's syndrome, hypogonadotrophic
      eunuchoidism)
   Acquired hypogonadism
    Viral orchitis
    Trauma
    Radiation
    Hepatic insufficiency
    Chronic pulmonary disease
    Chronic renal failure
    Granulomatous disease (especially leprosy)
   Testicular carcinoma
   Pituitary tumor, especially when associated with hyper-
      prolactinemia
   Pituitary insufficiency
Neurologic disease
   Anterior temporal lobe lesion
   Spinal cord disease (e.g., multiple sclerosis)

Loss of sensory input
  Diabetes mellitus
  Polyneuropathy
  Tabes dorsalis
  Dorsal root ganglia disease
Lesions of nervi erigentes
  Aortic bypass surgery
  Total prostatectomy
  Rectosigmoid surgery
Drugs
  Guanethidine
  Methyldopa
  Clonidine
  Spironolactone
  Reserpine
  Phenothiazines
  Imipramine
  Estrogens
  Heroin
  Methadone
  Lithium
Alcoholism
Vascular disease (e.g., Leriche syndrome)
Priapism
Penile disease
  Trauma
  Peyronie's disease

Reference

1. Walsh PC, Wilson JD: Disturbances of Sexual Function
    and Reproduction in Men. In general reference 1,
    p 229.

7-O. Menorrhagia and Nonmenstrual Vaginal Bleeding

Anovulatory bleeding
Abortion
Ectopic pregnancy
Carcinoma (endometrium, cervix, vagina)
Endometritis, vaginitis
Endometriosis
Fibroid tumors
Intrauterine device
Estrogen therapy, oral contraceptives
Bleeding diathesis (including oral anticoagulant therapy)
Hypothyroidism
Feminizing ovarian tumor
Acute exanthematous infectious disease
Stress

Reference

1. McArthur JW: Diseases of the Ovary. In general reference 1, p 1775.

8

Hematologic System

8-A. Microcytic Anemia

Hypochromic
Iron lack
  Chronic blood loss
  Pregnancy
  Dietary iron deficiency (especially infants, teenagers)
  Impaired absorption
    Subtotal gastrectomy
    Malabsorption syndromes
  Intravascular hemolysis
    Mechanical trauma (e.g., valve prosthesis, microan-
      giopathic hemolytic anemia)
    Paroxysmal nocturnal hemoglobinuria
  Hemodialysis
Hemoglobin abnormalities
  Thalassemia syndromes
  Hemoglobin Köln, Lepore, H, E
Blockade of heme synthesis
  Lead
  Isoniazid
  Pyrazinamide
Sideroblastic anemia, hereditary
  X-linked
  Autosomal recessive
Anemia of chronic disease
Familial

Normochromic
Hereditary spherocytosis
Spherocytosis of other causes

References
1. Fairbanks VF, Beutler E: Iron Deficiency. In general
   reference 20, p 363.
2. Valentine WN: Sideroblastic Anemias. In general reference 20, p 418.

8-B. Macrocytic (Megaloblastic) Anemia

Vitamin B$_{12}$ Deficiency
Inadequate dietary intake (rare)
Impaired absorption
  Inadequate intrinsic factor (IF)
    Pernicious anemia
    Gastrectomy, total or partial
    Gastric mucosal injury (e.g., lye ingestion)
    Anti-IF antibody in gastric juice
    Transplacental anti-IF antibody
    Congenital
      Absence of IF
      Nonfunctional IF antibody
  Malabsorption
    Sprue, tropical or nontropical
    Ileal resection
    Regional ileitis
    Infiltrative intestinal disease (e.g., lymphoma,
      leukemia, Whipple's disease, amyloidosis)
    Chronic pancreatitis
    Familial selective malabsorption
  Drugs
    Colchicine
    Para-aminosalicylic acid
    Neomycin
  Parasites, competition for B$_{12}$

Bacteria in blind loops, pouches, diverticula, anastomoses

Fish tapeworm infestation

Transcobalamin II deficiency

Folic Acid Deficiency

Inadequate dietary intake (especially alcoholics, infants)

Impaired absorption

Sprue, tropical or nontropical

Steatorrhea of other causes

Gastrectomy

Small-intestine resection or bypass

Infiltration of small intestine (e.g., leukemia, lymphoma, Whipple's disease, amyloidosis)

Scleroderma

Diabetes mellitus

Drugs (e.g., phenytoin, phenobarbital, oral contraceptives)

Increased requirements

Pregnancy

Infancy

Malignancy

Uremia

Skin diseases (e.g., exfoliative dermatitis, psoriasis)

Hyperactive hemopoiesis (e.g., hemolytic anemia)

Impaired metabolism

Alcohol

Dihydrofolate reductase inhibition

Methotrexate

Triamterene

Pyrimethamine

Dihydrofolate reductase deficiency

Other Causes

Sideroblastic anemia, acquired

Idiopathic, primary

Secondary

Drug-induced

Ethanol

Lead

Isoniazid

Chloramphenicol

Cycloserine

Antineoplastics

Neoplasm (especially multiple myeloma, lymphoma)

Inflammatory diseases (e.g., rheumatoid arthritis)

Hematologic disorders (e.g., myelofibrosis, hemolytic anemia)

Metabolic disorders (e.g., myxedema, uremia)

Drugs that impair metabolism
    Purine antagonists
        6-Mercaptopurine
        6-Thioguanine
        Azathioprine
    Pyrimidine antagonists
        5-Fluorouracil
        Cytosine arabinoside
        6-Azauridine
    Others
        Hydroxyurea
Inborn errors of metabolism
    Hereditary orotic aciduria
    Lesch-Nyhan syndrome
Other rare causes
    Vitamin C deficiency (scurvy)
    Pyridoxine-responsive megaloblastic anemia
    Thiamine-responsive megaloblastic anemia
    Refractory megaloblastic anemia
    Erythremic myelosis (di Guglielmo's syndrome)

References

1. Beck, WS: Vitamin B_{12} Deficiency. In general reference 20, p 307.
2. Beck WS: Folic Acid Deficiency. In general reference 20, p 334.
3. Beck WS: Megaloblastic Anemias Unresponsive to Vitamin B_{12} or Folic Acid. In general reference 20, p 356.
4. Babior BM, Bunn HF: Megaloblastic Anemias. In general reference 1, p 1518.

8-C. Normocytic Anemia

Associated with Increased Red Cell Production
Posthemorrhage
Hemolysis (see 8-D)

Associated with Decreased Red Cell Production
Bone marrow disorders
    Hypoplasia
        Aplastic anemia (see 8-F)
        Pure red cell aplasia

Infiltration of the bone marrow (see 8-F, "Myelophthisic
  disorders")
  Congenital dyserythropoietic anemias
Iron deficiency (early stages)
Anemia of chronic disorders
  Chronic infection
    Subacute bacterial endocarditis
    Osteomyelitis
    Chronic pyelonephritis
    Lung abscess
    Tuberculosis
    Chronic fungal infection
    Meningitis
    Pelvic inflammatory disease
  Chronic inflammation
    Rheumatoid arthritis
    Rheumatic fever
    Systemic lupus erythematosus
    Vasculitides (e.g., temporal arteritis)
    Sarcoidosis
    Regional enteritis
    Thermal burns
    Severe trauma
  Malignancy
    Carcinoma
    Lymphoma
    Leukemia
    Multiple myeloma
  Chronic renal insufficiency
  Chronic liver disease
  Endocrine disorders
    Hypothyroidism
    Adrenal insufficiency
    Hypogonadism
    Panhypopituitarism
    Hyperparathyroidism

Associated with Normal Red Cell Production
Dilutional anemia

References
1. Wintrobe MM, Lee GR, Boggs DR, et al: *Clinical
   Hematology.* Philadelphia: Lea & Febiger, 1974, p 693.
2. Erslev AJ: Anemia of Chronic Renal Failure; Anemia of
   Endocrine Disorders; Anemia of Chronic Disorders. In
   general reference 20, pp 288, 295, 434.
3. Bunn HF: Anemia Associated with Chronic Systemic
   Disorders. In general reference 1, p 1530.

8-D. Hemolytic Anemia

Hemolysis due to Extracellular Factors
Autoimmune agents
Warm antibodies (IgG, maximally active at 37°C)
  Idiopathic
  Secondary
    Malignancy or lymphoproliferative disorder
      Leukemia, especially chronic lymphocytic
      Lymphoma
      Multiple myeloma
      Thymoma
      Carcinoma (especially cervix, colon, uterus, kidney, lung)
    Infection
      Viral
        Infectious mononucleosis
        Rubeola
        Cytomegalovirus
        Herpes simplex
        Infectious hepatitis
      Bacterial, severe
        Bacteremia
        Pneumonia
        Meningitis
        Subacute bacterial endocarditis
      Mycobacterial
    Collagen-vascular disorders (especially systemic lupus erythematosus, rheumatoid arthritis, serum sickness)
    Gastrointestinal disorders (especially hepatitis, ulcerative colitis, pernicious anemia)
    Thyroid disorders (especially thyroiditis, hypothyroidism)
    Drug-induced
      Anti-inflammatory agents
        Indomethacin
        Phenylbutazone
        Phenacetin
      Anticonvulsants
        Phenytoin
        Mesantoin
      Antibiotics
        Penicillin
        Streptomycin
        Cephalosporins
        Isoniazid

      Para-aminosalicylic acid
      Rifampin
    Others
      Alpha methyldopa
      L-dopa
      Quinidine
      Quinine
      Chlorpropamide
      Methadone
      Chlorpromazine
      Chlordiazepoxide
Cold antibodies (IgM, maximally active at < 31°C)
  Idiopathic
  Secondary
    Viral infections
      Pneumonia
      Influenza
      Infectious mononucleosis
    Other infections
      Mycoplasma pneumonia
    Neoplasms
      Leukemia
      Lymphoma
      Carcinoma
  Paroxysmal cold hemoglobinuria (IgG)
Isoimmune hemolytic disease of the newborn (ABO or Rh
    incompatibility)
Congenital dyserythropoietic anemia (HEMPAS type)
Physical agents
Heat, thermal burns
Trauma
  March hemoglobinuria
  Cardiac prosthetic valves
  Microangiopathic anemia
Radiation
Animal and vegetable agents
Insect stings
Snakebites
Fava or castor beans
Infectious agents (nonimmune mechanism), especially:
Malaria
Leishmaniasis
Bartonellosis
Clostridium perfringens
Salmonella typhosa
Others
Chemical agents
Benzene

Toluene
Dinitrobenzene
Lead
Copper
Arsine
Sodium chlorate
Potassium chlorate
Hyperbaric oxygen
Water
  Freshwater drowning
  Intravenous distilled water
Miscellaneous
Hemolytic-uremic syndrome
Thrombotic thrombocytopenic purpura
Hypersplenism
Sarcoidosis
Wilson's disease
Hypophosphatemia

Hemolysis due to Intracellular Factors
Membrane abnormalities
  Hereditary spherocytosis
  Hereditary elliptocytosis
  Acanthocytosis (abetalipoproteinemia)
  Zieve's syndrome
  Paroxysmal nocturnal hemoglobinuria
Hemoglobinopathies
  Sickle cell disease
  Thalassemias
  Other abnormal hemoglobins
Enzyme deficiencies
  Disorders of anaerobic glycolysis (e.g., pyruvate-kinase
    deficiency)
  Disorders of the hexose monophosphate shunt (especially glucose 6-phosphate dehydrogenase deficiency)
  Congenital erythropoietic porphyria

References
1. General reference 20, pp 453–610.
2. Pirofsky B: *Auto-Immunization and the Auto-Immune Hemolytic Anemias.* Baltimore, Md.: Williams & Wilkins, 1969.
3. Cooper RA, Bunn HF: Hemolytic Anemias. In general reference 1, p 1533.

8-E. Drugs That Cause Hemolysis in Patients with G-6-PD Deficiency

Sulfonamides and sulfones
Other antibiotics
    Nitrofurantoin
    Chloramphenicol
    Nalidixic acid
    Para-aminosalicylic acid
Analgesics
    Phenacetin
    Acetanilid
    Acetylsalicylic acid*
Antimalarials
    Chloroquine
    Quinine
    Primaquine
    Pamaquine
Others
    Vitamin K (water-soluble)
    Probenecid
    Phenylhydrazine
    Quinidine
    Methylene blue*
    Ascorbic acid*

References

1. Beutler E: Glucose 6-phosphate Dehydrogenase Deficiency. In general reference 20, p 466.
2. Cooper RA, Bunn HF: Hemolytic Anemias. In general reference 1, p 1533.

*Only in large doses.

8-F. Pancytopenia

Pancytopenia with Hypocellular Marrow
Aplastic anemia
  Idiopathic
  Drugs, chemicals
    Common
      Cytotoxic agents
      Chloramphenicol
      Phenylbutazone
      Benzene
    More than 10 reported cases
      Acetazolamide
      Acetophenetidin
      Acetylsalicylic acid
      Chlorothiazide
      Chlorpheniramine
      Chlorpromazine
      Phenytoin
      Gold salts
      Meprobamate
      Penicillin
      Potassium perchlorate
      Prochlorperazine
      Streptomycin
      Sulfonamides
      Tolbutamide
  Radiation
  Infection
    Viral (especially hepatitis)
    Mycobacterial (especially miliary tuberculosis)
  Immune reaction (e.g., graft versus host reaction)
  Congenital aplastic anemia
  Others
    Systemic lupus erythematosus
    Pregnancy
    Pancreatitis
Myelophthisic disorders
  Aleukemic leukemia
  Lymphoma
  Multiple myeloma
  Metastatic carcinoma
  Myelofibrosis
  Gaucher's disease
  Osteopetrosis
  Miliary tuberculosis
Paroxysmal nocturnal hemoglobinuria

Pancytopenia with Normocellular Marrow
Idiopathic
Drug-induced (especially chloramphenicol, benzene, estrogens)
Overwhelming infection
Acute granulocytic leukemia
Hypersplenism
Sideroblastic anemia
Nutritional deficiency
    Vitamin B_{12}
    Folate
Congenital dyserythropoietic anemia
Sarcoidosis

References
1. Erslev AJ: Aplastic Anemia. In general reference 20, p 258.
2. Valentine WN: Pancytopenia with Cellular Marrow (Non-Sideroblastic). In general reference 20, p 431.
3. MM Wintrobe, GR Lee, DR Boggs, et al: *Clinical Hematology.* Philadelphia: Lea & Febiger, 1974, p 1741.

8-G. Polycythemia*

Spurious
Decreased plasma volume (especially severe dehydration, extensive burns, Addison's disease)
Stress erythrocytosis

Primary
Polycythemia vera

Secondary
Appropriate (associated with tissue hypoxia)
    Decreased arterial PO_2
        Altitude
        Pulmonary disease
        Alveolar hypoventilation
        Cyanotic congenital heart disease

*Increased red cell mass.

Normal arterial PO$_2$
   Hemoglobin abnormalities
      Carboxyhemoglobinemia (e.g., excessive cigarette
         smoking)
      Hemoglobinopathies (hemoglobins with increased
         affinity for oxygen)
      Methemoglobinemia
      Sulfhemoglobinemia
   Impaired oxygen delivery
      Chronic congestive heart failure
      Acquired cardiac valvular disease
   Tissue hypoxia of other causes (e.g., cobalt)
Inappropriate
   Renal disorders
      Renal vascular impairment
      Hydronephrosis
      Renal cyst
      Renal tumor
   Endocrine disorders
      Adrenal adenoma
         Cushing's syndrome
         Aldosterone-producing
      Pheochromocytoma
      Masculinizing ovarian tumor
      Androgen therapy
      Hypothalamic-pituitary disorders
   Hepatoma
   Cerebellar hemangioma
   Uterine myoma
   Benign familial erythrocytosis
   Erythrocytosis of the newborn

References

1. Erslev AJ: Secondary Polycythemia. In general reference 20, p 641.
2. Kraus S, Wasserman LR: Spurious (Relative) Polycythemia. In general reference 20, p 653.

8-H. Lymphadenopathy

Localized (Affecting Only Regional Nodes)
Infection
   Bacterial: Any local infection, especially:
      Streptococcal
      Staphylococcal
      Tularemia
      Syphilis, primary
      Tuberculosis
   Fungal: Any local infection (especially sporotrichosis,
      histoplasmosis)
   Viral (especially herpes zoster and herpes simplex, cat-
      scratch disease)
   Protozoal, especially leishmaniasis
   Rickettsial (especially rickettsialpox, scrub typhus)
   Chlamydial
      Trachoma
      Inclusion conjunctivitis
      Lymphogranuloma venereum
Malignancy
   Metastatic carcinoma
   Lymphoma
   Chronic myelogenous leukemia, blast crisis
Congenital abnormalities
   Lymphangiomas, cavernous or superficial
   Cystic hygroma
Local inflammation
   Reaction to antigen (e.g., vaccination)
   Chronic skin trauma
   Dermatitis
Other
   Mucocutaneous lymph node syndrome

Generalized (Enlargement of Cervical, Inguinal, and Axillary Nodes)*
Infection
   Bacterial (especially brucellosis, leptospirosis, tuber-
      culosis)
   Viral
      Common childhood viral illnesses
      Infectious mononucleosis
      Dengue fever
   Spirochetal
      Syphilis (congenital or secondary)
   Rickettsial, especially scrub typhus
   Protozoal, especially toxoplasmosis

Malignancy
    Leukemia
    Lymphoma
Hypersensitivity reactions
    Serum sickness
    Drug reaction, especially phenytoin (pseudolymphoma)
Endocrine disorders
    Hyperthyroidism
    Adrenal insufficiency
    Hypopituitarism
Autoimmune disorders
    Systemic lupus erythematosus
    Rheumatoid arthritis
    Dermatomyositis
    Autoimmune hemolytic anemias
Sarcoidosis
Other
    Agnogenic myeloid metaplasia
    Atypical lymph node hyperplasia
    Lipid storage diseases
    Exfoliative dermatitis
    Immunoblastic lymphadenopathy

References

1. Fefer A: Enlargement of the Lymph Nodes and Spleen.
   In general reference 1, p 279.
2. General reference 3, p 373.

*Most diseases causing generalized lymphadenopathy can also
cause localized lymph node enlargement.*

8-I. Splenomegaly

Idiopathic
Infection
    Bacterial, especially:
        Typhoid or paratyphoid fever
        Tularemia
        Subacute bacterial endocarditis
        Brucellosis

Mycobacterial (especially tuberculosis)
Viral (especially infectious mononucleosis,
    cytomegalovirus)
Rickettsial (especially Rocky Mountain spotted fever,
    murine typhus)
Fungal (especially histoplasmosis)
Spirochetal (especially secondary syphilis)
Parasitic
  Malaria
  Schistosomiasis
  Leishmaniasis
  Kala azar
  Toxoplasmosis
Congestion
  Portal hypertension
    Cirrhosis (see 6-Q)
    Banti's syndrome
  Thrombosis of portal or splenic vein
  Compression of portal or splenic vein
Hematologic disorders
  Nonmalignant
    Autoimmune hemolytic anemia
    Aplastic anemia
    Hemoglobinopathies
    Spherocytosis
    Thrombotic thrombocytopenic purpura
    Pseudolymphoma
  Malignant
    Lymphoma
    Leukemia
    Myeloid metaplasia
    Polycythemia vera
Autoimmune disorders
  Rheumatoid arthritis
  Felty's syndrome
  Systemic lupus erythematosus
  Serum sickness
Sarcoidosis
Infiltrative diseases
  Amyloidosis
  Lipid storage diseases
    Gaucher's disease
    Niemann-Pick disease
  Multifocal eosinophilic granuloma
  Letterer-Siwe disease
Splenic disorders
  Subcapsular hemorrhage

Splenic infarct
Splenic artery aneurysm
Splenic cyst (especially *Echinococcus*)
Splenic abscess
Splenic tumor
    Lymphangioma, hemangioma
    Metastatic (rare)

References
1. Fefer A: Enlargement of Lymph Nodes and Spleen. In general reference 1, p 279.
2. General reference 3, p 373.
3. Weinstein, IM: Lymph Node Enlargement and Splenomegaly. In general reference 20, p 950.

8-J. Granulocytopenia*

Infections
    Viral
        Influenza
        Infectious mononucleosis
        Rubeola
        Rubella
        Infectious hepatitis
        Chickenpox
        Smallpox
        Poliomyelitis
        Dengue fever
        Sandfly fever
    Bacterial
        Typhoid fever
        Paratyphoid fever
        Tularemia
        Brucellosis
        Psittacosis

*<1800 cells/mm³ in nonblacks, <1400 cells/mm³ in blacks.

Rickettsial
  Scrub typhus
Spirochetal
  Relapsing fever
  Kala azar
Protozoal
  Malaria
Other
  Bacteremia
  Miliary tuberculosis
  Overwhelming infection
Hematopoietic disorders
  Aleukemic leukemia
  Preleukemia
  Megaloblastic anemias
  Aplastic anemia
  Hypersplenism (see 8-I)
    Primary or secondary (especially Felty's syndrome)
  Myelophthisic disorders
  Chronic idiopathic neutropenia
  Pseudoneutropenia
Chemotherapy for malignancy
Idiosyncratic drug reactions (commonly used drugs)
  Antibiotics
    Sulfonamides
    Penicillin
    Chloramphenicol
    Cephalothin
    Gentamicin
    Streptomycin
    Isoniazid
  Antihistamines (e.g., pyribenzamine)
  Analgesics, anti-inflammatory agents
    Phenacetin
    Antipyrine
    Phenylbutazone
    Indomethacin
  Anticonvulsants
    Phenytoin
    Carbamazepine
    Mephenytoin
    Primidone
    Trimethadione
  Antithyroid agents
    Propylthiouracil
    Carbamazepine
    Methimazole
  Diuretics
    Chlorthalidone

Hydrochlorthiazide
Acetazolamide
Ethacrynic acid
Cardiac drugs
Procainamide
Quinidine
Alpha methyldopa
Propranolol
Phenothiazines
Other neuropharmacologic agents
Diazepam
Imipramine
L-dopa
Meprobamate
Barbiturates
Oral hypoglycemics
Others
Allopurinol
Ethanol
Ionizing radiation
Anaphylaxis
Severe malnutrition
Others
Systemic lupus erythematosus
Familial neutropenia
Cyclic neutropenia

References
1. Finch SC: Granulocytopenia. In general reference 20, p 717.
2. General reference 19, p 759.

8-K. Granulocytosis*

Reactive Granulocytosis
Infection
    Bacterial (primarily)
    Fungal
    Rickettsial
    Viral
    Spirochetal
    Parasitic
Physical stimuli
    Exercise
    Pain, trauma
    Extreme temperature
    Smoking
    Ovulation, pregnancy
    Seizures
Inflammation, acute and chronic
Neoplasm
Tissue necrosis
    Myocardial infarction
    Gangrene
    Burns
Drugs, toxins, especially:
    Corticosteroids
    Epinephrine
    Lithium
    Endotoxin
    Histamine
Hematologic disorders
    Hemorrhage
    Postsplenectomy, functional asplenia
    Megaloblastic anemia during therapy
    Recovery from agranulocytosis
    Hemolytic anemia
Metabolic disorders
    Acidosis
    Cushing's syndrome
    Eclampsia
    Thyroid storm

Autonomous Granulocytosis
Leukemia, especially chronic myelocytic
Polycythemia vera

*>6500 cells/mm^3.

Myeloid metaplasia
Chronic idiopathic leukocytosis
Cyclic leukocytosis

Hereditary Disorders
Hereditary neutrophilic leukemoid reaction
Familial cold urticaria

References
1. Finch SC: Granulocytosis. In general reference 20, p 746.
2. General reference 19, p 759.

8-L. Lymphocytosis*

Infections
  Viral
    Infectious mononucleosis
    Infectious lymphocytosis
    Cytomegalovirus infection
    Mumps
    Rubella
    Chickenpox
    Viral hepatitis
  Bacterial
    Pertussis
    Brucellosis
    Tuberculosis
  Spirochetal
    Syphilis, secondary and congenital
  Protozoan
    Toxoplasmosis
Hematologic disorders
  Lymphocytic leukemia
  Leukosarcoma
  Non-Hodgkin's lymphoma
Drugs (rare)
  Phenytoin
  p-Aminosalicylic acid

*>4000 cells/mm³.

Miscellaneous
    Thyrotoxicosis
    Adrenal insufficiency
    Post-cardiopulmonary-bypass syndrome
    Hypersensitivity reactions (rare)

References

1. Cassileth PA: Lymphocytosis. In general reference 20, p 968.
2. General reference 19, p 759.

8-M. Monocytosis*

Infections
    Subacute bacterial endocarditis
    Tuberculosis
    Syphilis: Primary, secondary, congenital
    Brucellosis
    Typhoid fever
    Rickettsial infections
    Kala azar
    Trypanosomiasis
    Leishmaniasis
    Malaria
Hematologic disorders
    Preleukemia
    Leukemia: Monocytic, lymphocytic, granulocytic
    Lymphoma, Hodgkin's and non-Hodgkin's
    Polycythemia vera
    Myeloid metaplasia
    Multiple myeloma
    Neutropenia
        Agranulocytosis of various causes (see 8-J)

*>750 cells/mm³.

Cyclic neutropenia
Chronic granulocytopenia of childhood
Familial neutropenia
Hemolytic anemias
Hypochromic anemias
Idiopathic thrombocytopenic purpura
Postsplenectomy
Autoimmune diseases
Rheumatoid arthritis
Systemic lupus erythematosus
Temporal arteritis
Polyarteritis nodosa
Myositis
Malignancy
Approximately 60% of nonhematologic malignancies
Gastrointestinal disorders
Sprue
Ulcerative colitis
Regional enteritis
Miscellaneous
Fever of unknown origin
Sarcoidosis
Hand-Schüller-Christian disease

References

1. Cassileth PA: Monocytosis. In general reference 20, p 974.
2. General reference 19, p 759.

8-N. Eosinophilia*

Drug reactions
  Allergic
  Idiosyncratic
    Erythromycin estolate
    Sulfonamides
    p-Aminosalicylic acid
    Nitrofurantoin
    Chlorpropamide
    Imipramine
    Procarbazine
    Methotrexate
Parasitic infections
  Protozoans (especially toxicariasis, toxoplasmosis, amebiasis)
  Metazoans (especially trichinosis, filariasis, schistosomiasis)
  Arthropods (especially scabies, *Tunga penetrans* [chiggers])
Allergic disorders
  Allergic rhinitis (hay fever)
  Asthma
  Bronchopulmonary aspergillosis
  Urticaria
  Angioneurotic edema
  Serum sickness
  Food allergy
  Hypersensitivity angiitis
  Allergic eczema
  Erythema multiforme
  Erythema neonatorum
  Dermatitis herpetiformis
Chronic skin disorders
  Psoriasis
  Pruritus secondary to jaundice
  Exfoliative dermatitis
  Pityriasis rosea
  Leprosy
  Ichthyosis
  Pemphigus vulgaris
  Facial granulomas
Hematopoietic disorders
  Lymphoma, especially Hodgkin's
  Eosinophilic leukemoid reaction

*>450 cells/mm^3.

Postsplenectomy
Chronic myelogenous leukemia
Polycythemia vera
Idiopathic thrombocytopenic purpura
Hyperleukocytosis with eosinophilia in children
Familial histiocytosis
Malignant disorders
  Carcinomatosis
  Mycosis fungoides
  Melanoma
  Eosinophilic granuloma
Autoimmune disorders
  Rheumatoid disease
  Polyarteritis nodosa
  Granulomatous vasculitis
  Dermatomyositis
  Henoch-Schönlein purpura
Hypereosinophilic syndromes
  Loeffler's disease
  Loeffler's fibroplastic endocarditis
  Eosinophilic pneumonia
Gastrointestinal disorders
  Eosinophilic gastroenteritis
  Eosinophilic peritonitis
  Ulcerative colitis
  Regional enteritis
Others
  Sarcoidosis
  Post–radiation therapy, especially to abdomen
  Chronic renal disease
  Peritoneal dialysis
  Adrenal insufficiency
  Magnesium deficiency
  Scarlet fever
  Tuberculous lymphadenitis
  Coccidioidomycosis
Familial or hereditary eosinophilia

References

1. Finch SC: Granulocytosis. In general reference 20, p 746.
2. General reference 19, p 759.
3. Dale DC: Abnormalities of Leukocytes. In general reference 1, p 290.

8-O. Thrombocytopenia*

Increased Destruction
Immune mechanisms
  Idiopathic autoimmune thrombocytopenic purpura
  Drugs (partial list)
    Quinidine
    Quinine
    Digitalis
    p-Aminosalicylic acid
    Methyldopa
    Rifampin
    Ethchlorvynol
    Thiazides
    Gold salts
    Chloroquine
    Sulfonamides
    Meprobamate
    Phenylbutazone
    Stibophen
  Posttransfusion purpura
  Allergy, anaphylaxis
  Antilymphocyte globulin
  Congenital
    Associated with maternal idiopathic thrombocytopenic purpura
    Associated with maternal drug ingestion
    Isoimmune neonatal thrombocytopenia
  Others
    Sarcoidosis
    Lymphoma
    Chronic lymphocytic lymphoma
    Systemic lupus erythematosus
    Scleroderma
    Hashimoto's thyroiditis
    Thyrotoxicosis
    Carcinomatosis
Nonimmune mechanisms
  Infections
    Bacterial
      Severe gram-positive or gram-negative infections
      Typhoid fever
      Diphtheria
    Fungal (especially histoplasmosis)

*<150,000 platelets/mm³.

    Rickettsial (especially scrub typhus, Rocky Mountain
        spotted fever)
    Parasitic (especially malaria, trypanosomiasis)
    Viral, especially:
        Mumps
        Varicella
        Cytomegalovirus
        Infectious mononucleosis
Drugs, direct toxicity
    Ristocetin
    Heparin
Mechanical injury
    Cardiac valvular disease
        Aortic stenosis
        Prosthetic valves
    Extracorporeal circulation
Congenital and neonatal
    Erythroblastosis fetalis
    Thrombocytopenia of prematurity
    Renal vein thrombosis
    Indwelling umbilical artery catheter
    Cavernous hemangioma
Other
    Disseminated intravascular coagulation
    Burns
    Fat embolism
    Thrombotic thrombocytopenic purpura
    Hemolytic-uremic syndrome
    Transplant rejection
    Primary pulmonary hypertension
    Hemangioma
    Splenic hamartoma

Decreased Production
Aplastic anemia (see 8-F)
Aplasia of megakaryocytes
Marrow infiltration
    Lymphoma
    Leukemia
    Multiple myeloma
    Carcinoma
    Myelofibrosis
    Gaucher's disease
    Osteopetrosis
    Miliary tuberculosis
Ionizing radiation
Myelosuppressive drugs, especially:
    Cytosine arabinoside

    Cyclophosphamide
    Busulfan
    Methotrexate
    6-Mercaptopurine
Drugs, other
    Thiazides
    Alcohol
    Estrogen
Cyclic thrombocytopenia
Nutritional deficiency
    Folate
    Vitamin B_{12}
    Iron
Viral infections, especially:
    Influenza
    Rubella
    Rubeola
    Infectious mononucleosis
    Thai hemorrhagic fever
    Dengue fever
Paroxysmal nocturnal hemoglobinuria
Hereditary diseases (especially Wiskott-Aldrich syndrome,
    May-Hegglin anomaly)
Congenital causes
    Fanconi's anemia
    Amegakaryocytic thrombocytopenia with congenital
        malformations
    Congenital rubella or cytomegalovirus infection
    Maternal thiazide ingestion
    Congenital deficiency of thrombopoietin
    Bilateral aplasia of the radius

Sequestration
Hypersplenism
Hypothermia
Trauma
Venous stasis
Adult respiratory distress syndrome

Platelet Loss
Severe hemorrhage (especially if requiring multiple
    transfusions of bank blood)
Exchange transfusion
Extracorporeal circulation

Pseudothrombocytopenia
Cold agglutinins
Platelet-granulocyte rosettes

References
1. Aster RH: Disorders of Hemostasis: Quantitative Platelet Disorders. In general reference 20, p 1317.
2. Nossel HL: Platelet Disorders. In general reference 1, p 1555.

8-P. Thrombocytosis*

Primary
Essential thrombocythemia
Polycythemia vera
Chronic granulocytic leukemia
Idiopathic myelofibrosis

Secondary
Malignancy (especially carcinoma, lymphoma)
Inflammatory disease
  Acute
    Recovery from acute infection
  Chronic
    Rheumatoid arthritis
    Acute rheumatic fever
    Tuberculosis
    Cirrhosis
    Sarcoidosis
    Osteomyelitis
    Slowly resolving bacterial infection
    Ulcerative colitis
    Regional enteritis
    Polyarteritis nodosa
    Wegener's granulomatosis
Acute hemorrhage
Iron deficiency
Hemolytic anemia
Postoperative
  Splenectomy
  Other surgery
Postexercise

Drugs
  Vincristine
  Epinephrine
Recovery from thrombocytopenia
  Recovery from cytotoxic or immunosuppressive drugs
  Therapy of megaloblastic anemia
  Rebound from chronic ethanol ingestion

References
1. Williams WJ: Thrombocytosis. In general reference 20, p 1364.
2. General reference 19, p 883.

*>400,000 platelets/mm³.

8-Q. Disorders of Hemostasis

Platelet Disorders
Abnormal numbers of platelets
  Thrombocytopenia (see 8-O)
  Thrombocytosis (see 8-P)
Abnormal platelet function
  Congenital
    Impaired platelet adhesion
      Bernard-Soulier (giant-platelet) syndrome
      von Willebrand's disease
    Impaired platelet aggregation
      Thrombasthenia (Glanzmann's disease)
    Abnormal platelet factor 3
    Agranular platelets
    Platelet abnormalities with other congenital defects,
        especially:
      Wiskott-Aldrich syndrome
      Connective-tissue disorders
        Ehlers-Danlos syndrome
        Pseudoxanthoma elasticum
        Osteogenesis imperfecta

Acquired
  Uremia
  Myeloproliferative disorders
    Essential thrombocytopenia
    Polycythemia vera
    Myeloid metaplasia
    Acute leukemia
    Chronic granulocytic leukemia
  Dysproteinemias (especially macroglobulinemia,
      multiple myeloma)
  Liver disease
  Idiopathic thrombocytopenic purpura
  Drug-induced
    Acetylsalicylic acid
    Anesthetics, local and general
    Carbenicillin
    Dextran
    Dipyridamole
    Ethanol
    Hydroxyethyl starch
    Sulfinpyrazone

Vascular Disorders
Nonthrombocytopenic purpura
  Nonallergic purpura
    Purpura simplex
    Mechanical purpura
    Senile purpura
    Cushing's disease
    Connective-tissue disorders
      Pseudoxanthoma elasticum
      Ehlers-Danlos syndrome
      Marfan's syndrome
      Osteogenesis imperfecta
    Scurvy
    Dysproteinemias
      Cryoglobulinemia
      Cryofibrinogenemia
      Multiple myeloma
      Amyloidosis
      Benign hyperglobulinemia
    Infections
      Bacterial
        Bacteremia, gram-positive or gram-negative
          (especially meningococcemia)
        Typhoid fever
        Subacute bacterial endocarditis
      Viral
      Rickettsial

Drug-induced (especially penicillin, sulfonamides)
Autoerythrocyte sensitivity
Allergic purpura (e.g., Henoch-Schönlein purpura)
Hereditary hemorrhagic telangiectasia

Coagulation Disorders
Congenital
  Deficiency of blood coagulation factors (in approximate
      order of clinical incidence)
    Factor VIII (hemophilia A)
    Factor IX (hemophilia B)
    Factor XI
    Factor V
    Factor VII
    Factor X
    Factor II
  Disorders of fibrinogen
    Afibrinogenemia
    Hypofibrinogenemia
    Dysfibrinogenemia
  Combined platelet and coagulation factor abnormalities
    von Willebrand's disease
Acquired
  Vitamin K deficiency
    Hemorrhagic disease of the newborn
    Malabsorption states
    Oral anticoagulants
  Liver disease
  Amyloidosis
  Nephrotic syndrome
  Gaucher's disease
  Systemic lupus erythematosus
  Circulating anticoagulants
  Disseminated intravascular coagulation

References
1. General reference 20, pp 1311–1494.
2. Nossel HL: Clotting Disorders. In general reference 1,
  p 1555.

9
Infectious Disease

9-A. Fever of Unknown Origin in the United States*

Infection†
Bacterial
  Sinusitis
  Bacterial endocarditis
  Osteomyelitis
  Upper abdominal cause, e.g.:
    Cholangitis
    Cholecystitis
    Empyema of gallbladder
    Pancreatic, hepatic, subphrenic abscess
  Lower abdominal cause, e.g.:
    Appendiceal abscess
    Diverticulitis
    Pelvic inflammatory disease or abscess
    Perirectal abscess
    Peritonitis
  Urinary tract cause, e.g.:
    Perinephric, intrarenal, or prostatic abscess
    Pyelonephritis (rare)
    Ureteral obstruction

*Defined as temperature of > 38.3°C daily for 2 to 3 weeks, with cause undiagnosed despite 1 week of intensive studies in hospital.

Bacteremia without primary focus, especially:
- Meningococcemia
- Gonococcemia
- Salmonellosis
- Listeriosis
- Brucellosis
- Yersiniosis
- Tularemia
- Leptospirosis
- Syphilis
Tuberculosis
Viral (e.g., Epstein-Barr virus [infectious mononucleosis], coxsackie B, cytomegalovirus)
Chlamydial, rickettsial (e.g., psittacosis, Q fever)
Parasitic, protozoan, especially:
- Amebiasis
- Trichinosis
- Malaria
- Toxoplasmosis
Fungal, especially:
- Histoplasmosis
- Blastomycosis
- Cryptococcosis
- Coccidioidomycosis

Malignancy†
Leukemia, lymphoma
Solid tumor, especially carcinoma of:
- Kidney
- Lung
- Pancreas
- Liver
- Colon
Atrial myxoma

Collagen-Vascular Disease†
Lupus erythematosus
Rheumatoid arthritis
Rheumatic fever
Polyarteritis nodosa, hypersensitivity vasculitis
Wegener's granulomatosis
Temporal arteritis

Drugs
Antibiotics, especially:
- Penicillins
- Cephalosporins
- Sulfonamides
- Amphotericin B

Allopurinol
Phenytoin
Barbiturates
Iodides
Methyldopa
Procainamide
Quinidine
Propylthiouracil

Other
Pulmonary emboli, multiple
Thrombophlebitis
Sarcoidosis
Hepatitis, granulomatous or alcoholic
Inflammatory bowel disease
Whipple's disease
Thyroiditis
Thyrotoxicosis
Trauma with hematoma in enclosed space (e.g.,
    perisplenic, perivesical)
Myelofibrosis
Hemolytic states
Dissecting aneurysm
Fabry's disease
Familial Mediterranean fever
Gout
Addison's disease
Weber-Christian disease
Cyclic neutropenia
Thermoregulatory disorders
Factitious fever
Habitual hyperthermia

References

1. Petersdorf RG: Chills and Fever. In general reference
   1, p 60.
2. Jacoby GA, Swartz MN: Current Concepts: Fever of
   Undetermined Origin. *N Engl J Med* 289:1407, 1973.

†Infection, malignancy, and collagen-vascular disease ultimately
account for about 75% of fevers of unknown origin.

9-B. Most Common Organisms Causing Specific Infections

Skin infection	
Burns	*Staphylococcus aureus, Streptococcus pyogenes, Pseudomonas,* and other gram-negative bacilli
Decubiti	*Staph. aureus,* group A *Strep.,* anaerobic *Strep., Escherichia coli,* and other gram-negative bacilli
Traumatic and surgical wounds	*Staph. aureus,* group A *Strep.,* anaerobic *Strep.,* clostridia, gram-negative bacilli
Osteomyelitis	*Staph. aureus, Salmonella* and other gram-negative bacilli, group A *Strep.*
Arthritis, septic	*Staph. aureus,* pneumococcus, group A *Strep., Neisseria gonorrhoeae,* gram-negative bacilli (especially *E. coli, Salmonella, Pseudomonas*), *N. meningitidis*
Meningitis	Viruses, pneumococcus, *Haemophilus influenzae, N. meningitidis,* gram-negative bacilli, *Staph. aureus* and epidermidis, group A *Strep.*
Conjunctivitis, keratitis	Herpes and other viruses, pneumococcus, group A *Strep., Staph. aureus, Neisseria* species, *Pseudomonas* and other gram-negative bacilli, *H. aegyptius, Chlamydia, Moraxella lacunata*
Sinusitis	Pneumococcus, group A *Strep., Staph. aureus, H. influenzae, Klebsiella,* and other gram-negative bacilli

Pharyngitis	Respiratory viruses, group A *Strep.*, *H. influenzae* or *parainfluenzae*, *N. gonorrhoeae* or *meningitidis*
Laryngitis, tracheitis, bronchitis	Respiratory viruses, pneumococcus, *H. influenzae*, group A *Strep.*
Pleuritis	*Staph. aureus*, pneumococcus, *H. influenzae*, gram-negative bacilli, anaerobic *Strep.*, *Bacteroides*, *Mycobacterium tuberculosis*
Pneumonia	Respiratory viruses, *Mycoplasma pneumoniae*, pneumococcus, anaerobic bacteria, *H. influenzae*, *Staph. aureus*, *Klebsiella* and other gram-negative bacilli, *Legionella pneumophila*
Lung abscess	Anaerobic bacteria, *Klebsiella* and other gram-negative bacilli, *Staph. aureus*, group A *Strep.*
Endocarditis	
Subacute	*Strep. viridans*, enterococcus, other *Streptococci*, *Staph. aureus* and epidermidis, gram-negative bacilli
Acute	*Staph. aureus* and *epidermidis*, pneumococcus, group A *Strep.*, gram-negative bacilli, *Candida albicans* and other fungi
Gastroenteritis	Enteric viruses, *E. coli*, *Salmonella*, *Shigella*, *Campylobacter*
Peritonitis	*E. coli* and other gram-negative bacilli, enterococcus, *Bacteroides*, anaerobic *Strep.*, clostridia, pneumococcus

Urinary tract infection

Cystitis, pyelonephritis — *E. coli, Klebsiella, Enterobacter, Proteus,* and other gram-negative bacilli, enterococcus

Urethritis — *N. gonorrhoeae, Chlamydia, Trichomonas*

Vaginitis — *Trichomonas vaginalis, C. albicans,* group A *Strep., H. vaginalis, Treponema pallidum*

Pelvic inflammatory disease — *N. gonorrhoeae, E. coli* and other gram-negative bacilli, *Bacteroides,* anaerobic *Strep.,* enterococcus, clostridia

Salpingitis — *N. gonorrhoeae, E. coli* and other gram-negative bacilli, anaerobic *Strep., Bacteroides, C. trachomatis*

Epididymitis — *E. coli, Pseudomonas* and other gram-negative bacilli, *N. gonorrhoeae, C. trachomatis, M. tuberculosis*

Prostatitis — Gram-negative bacilli, *N. gonorrhoeae, Staph. aureus*

Septicemia — *E. coli* and other gram-negative bacilli, *Staph. aureus* and *epidermidis,* pneumococcus, *Bacteroides,* group A *Strep.,* enterococcus

References

1. General reference 1.
2. *Handbook of Antimicrobial Therapy.* New Rochelle, N.Y.: The Medical Letter, 1980, pp 9–11.

9-C. Antimicrobial Drugs of Choice

Gram-Positive Cocci	Drugs
Streptococcus pyogenes (group A)	Penicillin, erythromycin, cephalosporin
Strep. pneumoniae (pneumococcus)	Penicillin, cephalosporin, erythromycin, chloramphenicol, vancomycin
Enterococcus (group D *Strep.*)	Ampicillin or penicillin G or vancomycin, with or without amino-glycoside, erythromycin
Strep. viridans	Penicillin G or cephalosporin or vancomycin, with or without amino-glycoside
Strep., anaerobic (e.g., peptococcus, peptostreptococcus)	Penicillin G, erythromycin, clindamycin, chloramphenicol, cephalo-sporin
Staph. aureus	Penicillin or penicillinase-resistant penicillin, cephalosporin, clindamy-cin, vancomycin (with or without gentamicin or tobramycin for en-docarditis)
Staph. epidermidis	Penicillinase-resistant penicillin or cephalosporin or vancomycin, with or without gentamicin or tobramycin
Gram-Negative Cocci	
Neisseria gonorrhoeae (see also 3-D)	Penicillin G, ampicillin, amoxicillin, spectinomycin, tetracycline, erythro-mycin
N. meningitidis	Penicillin G, chloramphenicol, sulfonamide

Gram-Negative Bacilli	
Haemophilus influenzae	
Life-threatening infections	Chloramphenicol, ampicillin
Other	Ampicillin or amoxicillin, cefamandole, cefaclor, trimethoprim-sulfamethoxazole
Escherichia coli	Ampicillin, cephalosporin, gentamicin, tobramycin, amikacin, carbenicillin or ticarcillin, trimethoprim-sulfamethoxazole
Klebsiella pneumoniae	Aminoglycosides (especially gentamicin, tobramycin, amikacin) with or without cephalosporin, chloramphenicol
Enterobacter	Aminoglycosides (especially gentamicin, tobramycin, amikacin), carbenicillin or ticarcillin, chloramphenicol, tetracycline
Proteus mirabilis	Ampicillin, cephalosporin, aminoglycosides (especially gentamicin, tobramycin, amikacin), carbenicillin or ticarcillin, trimethoprim-sulfamethoxazole
Proteus, other	Aminoglycosides (especially amikacin, gentamicin, tobramycin), carbenicillin or ticarcillin, tetracycline, trimethoprim-sulfamethoxazole, cefoxitin, chloramphenicol
Providencia	Aminoglycosides (especially amikacin, gentamicin, tobramycin), carbenicillin or ticarcillin, trimethoprim-sulfamethoxazole, cefoxitin
Serratia	Aminoglycosides (especially amikacin) with or without carbenicillin or ticarcillin, trimethoprim-sulfamethoxazole, chloramphenicol

Pseudomonas aeruginosa	
Urinary tract infection	Carbenicillin or ticarcillin, gentamicin, tobramycin, amikacin
Other	Gentamicin or tobramycin or amikacin plus carbenicillin or ticarcillin
Salmonella typhosa	Chloramphenicol, ampicillin, amoxicillin, trimethoprim-sulfamethoxazole
Salmonella, other	Ampicillin or amoxicillin, chloramphenicol, trimethoprim-sulfamethoxazole
Shigella	Tetracycline, ampicillin, trimethoprim-sulfamethoxazole, nalidixic acid
Bacteroides fragilis	Clindamycin, chloramphenicol, metronidazole, cefoxitin
Brucella	Tetracycline with or without streptomycin, or gentamicin with or without sulfadiazine
Bordetella pertussis	Erythromycin, tetracycline, chloramphenicol
Acinetobacter	Aminoglycosides (especially gentamicin, tobramycin, amikacin) plus carbenicillin, minocycline, trimethoprim-sulfamethoxazole
Legionella pneumophila	Erythromycin, tetracycline, with or without rifampin
Gram-Positive Bacilli	
Listeria monocytogenes	Penicillin or ampicillin with or without aminoglycoside, tetracycline, erythromycin, chloramphenicol
Clostridium perfringens	Penicillin G, chloramphenicol, clindamycin

Gram-Positive Bacilli

C. tetani	Penicillin G, tetracycline, cephalosporin
Bacillus anthracis	Penicillin G, erythromycin, tetracycline, chloramphenicol

Miscellaneous Bacteria

Mycobacterium tuberculosis	Isoniazid and rifampin, ethambutol, streptomycin, PAS, pyrazinamide
Atypical mycobacteria	Isoniazid and rifampin with or without ethambutol, streptomycin, ethionamide, cycloserine, pyrazinamide, viomycin, or erythromycin
Actinomyces	Penicillin G, tetracycline, erythromycin, clindamycin
Nocardia	Sulfonamide with or without ampicillin, erythromycin, minocycline, or cycloserine
Treponema pallidum	Penicillin G, tetracycline, erythromycin, cephalosporin
Leptospira	Penicillin G, tetracycline

Fungi

Aspergillus	Amphotericin B with or without flucytosine or rifampin
Blastomyces dermatitidis	Amphotericin B, hydroxystilbamidine
Candida albicans	Amphotericin B with or without flucytosine (topical: nystatin, amphotericin B, miconazole, clotrimazole, ketoconazole)

Coccidioides immitis	Amphotericin B, miconazole
Cryptococcus neoformans	Amphotericin B with or without flucytosine
Histoplasma capsulatum	Amphotericin B
Sporothrix schenckii	Iodide (topical), amphotericin B

Others

Mycoplasma pneumoniae	Erythromycin, tetracycline
Rickettsia	Tetracycline, chloramphenicol
Chlamydia trachomatis	Tetracycline (especially doxycycline), sulfonamide
Herpes simplex	Adenine arabinoside (vidarabine), idoxuridine (topical, for keratitis only)
Pneumocystis carinii	Trimethoprim-sulfamethoxazole, pentamidine
Toxoplasma gondii	Pyrimethamine plus sulfonamide, clindamycin
Giardia lamblia	Quinacrine, metronidazole, furazolidone
Trichomonas vaginalis	Metronidazole

References

1. General reference 21.
2. *Handbook of Antimicrobial Therapy.* New Rochelle, N.Y.: The Medical Letter, 1980, pp 15–21.

9-D. VDRL, Biological False Positive

Infection
Spirochetal
  Yaws
  Pinta
  Bejel
  Leptospirosis
  Relapsing fever
  Rat-bite fever
Bacterial
  Pneumococcal pneumonia
  Scarlet fever
  Subacute bacterial endocarditis
  Tuberculosis
  Leprosy
  Chancroid
Viral
  Measles
  Varicella
  Vaccinia
  Hepatitis
  Infectious mononucleosis
  Postimmunization
Mycoplasmal
Chlamydial (lymphogranuloma venereum)
Rickettsial (typhus)
Protozoal (malaria, sleeping sickness)
Filarial
Fungal (coccidioidomycosis)

Noninfectious Causes
Aging
Pregnancy
Drug addiction
Collagen-vascular disease (especially lupus
    erythematosus, rheumatoid arthritis)
Serum sickness
Thyroiditis
Other hypergammaglobulinemic states
Blood transfusion

References
1. Holmes KK: Syphilis. In general reference 1, p 716.
2. Tramont EC: *Treponema Pallidum* (Syphilis). In general
   reference 21, p 1280.

10
Integument

10-A. Alopecia

Nonscarring
Pattern baldness
Traction
Drugs
   Cytotoxic agents
   Oral contraceptives
   Thallium
   Bismuth
   Borax
   Heparin, coumarin anticoagulants
   Ethionamide
   Vitamin A (excess)
   Thiouracil
Febrile illness, childbirth, other stressful states
Cutaneous disease (e.g., seborrheic dermatitis, eczema,
    psoriasis)
Cosmetics, other local irritants
Hypothyroidism
Hypopituitarism
Syphilis, secondary
Nutritional deficiency states (kwashiorkor, marasmus,
    iron deficiency)
Alopecia areata
Hereditary
Congenital

Scarring

Physical or chemical agents
  Burns
  Freezing
  Mechanical trauma
  Acid, alkali
  Radiation
Infection
  Bacterial (including pyogenic infection, tertiary
      syphilis, leprosy)
  Fungal (e.g., ringworm)
  Viral (especially varicella-zoster, variola)
  Protozoal
Systemic or discoid lupus erythematosus
Scleroderma
Sarcoidosis
Lichen planus
Epidermal nevi
Neoplasm
  Basal cell carcinoma
  Metastatic carcinoma
  Lymphoma
Congenital

Reference

1. Munro DD, Darley CR: Hair. In general reference 22,
   p 395.

10-B. Erythema Multiforme

Infections
  Viral (especially herpes)
  Bacterial
  Mycoplasmal
  Fungal
  Parasitic (*Trichomonas*)
Durgs, toxins
  Antibiotics (especially penicillin, sulfonamides,
      tetracyclines)
  Arsenic, mercury, gold
  Antihistamines
  Barbiturates
  Chlorpropamide
  Corticosteroids
  Phenytoin
  Codeine
  Hydralazine
  Salicylates
  Thiazides
  Quinine
  Phenylbutazone
Neoplasms and hematologic disorders
  Lymphoma
  Leukemia
  Carcinoma
  Multiple myeloma
  Polycythemia vera
Physical factors (radiation, sunlight, cold)
Collagen-vascular disease
  Systemic lupus erythematosus
  Dermatomyositis
  Rheumatoid arthritis
  Polyarteritis nodosa
  Wegener's granulomatosis
Menstruation, pregnancy
Reiter's syndrome
Idiopathic

Reference
1. Elias PM, Fritsch PO: Erythema Multiforme. In general
   reference 22, p 295.

10-C. Erythema Nodosum

Infection
  Beta streptococci
  Tuberculosis
  Histoplasmosis
  Coccidioidomycosis
  Blastomycosis
  Psittacosis
  Yersinia
  Trichophyton
  Lymphogranuloma venereum
  Chancroid
  Leprosy
  Cat-scratch fever
  Diphtheria
  Meningococcemia
Sarcoidosis
Behçet's disease
Lupus erythematosus
Rheumatic fever
Drugs
  Penicillins
  Tetracyclines
  Sulfonamides
  Halides
  Oral contraceptives
Inflammatory bowel disease
Idiopathic

Reference
1. Fitzpatrick TB, Haynes HA: Skin Lesions of General Medical Significance. In general reference 1, p 238.

10-D. Generalized Maculopapular Eruption

Drugs (especially antibiotics)
Infections
  Viral
    Rubeola
    Rubella
    Roseola
    Erythema infectiosum
    Infectious mononucleosis
    Cytomegalovirus
    Hepatitis B
    Other viruses (including adeno-, entero-, reo-, arbo-, rhabdovirus)
    Live-virus vaccine (e.g., measles)
  Bacterial, pyogenic
    Scarlet fever, other *Streptococcus* or *Staphylococcus* infection
    Pseudomonas septicemia
  Other
    Typhoid fever
    Syphillis, secondary
    Leptospirosis
    Rat-bite fever
    Rickettsial infection (e.g., Rocky Mountain spotted fever, murine typhus)
    Psittacosis
    Toxoplasmosis
    Trichinosis
Systemic lupus erythematosus
Dermatomyositis
Sarcoidosis
Erythema multiforme
Erythema marginatum
Pityriasis rosea

Reference
1. General reference 22.

10-E. Petechiae and Purpura

Intravascular Causes
Thrombocytopenia (see 8-O)
  Drugs, especially:
    Cytotoxic agents
    Quinidine
    Quinine
    Aspirin
    Phenytoin
    Phenylbutazone
    Indomethacin
    Gold
  Disseminated intravascular coagulation
    Overwhelming infection
      Bacterial infection (especially meningococcal,
        gonococcal, staphylococcal, gram-negative)
      Viral infection (especially entero-, arbo-,
        adenovirus)
      Rickettsial infection (Rocky Mountain spotted fever,
        louse-borne typhus)
      Miliary tuberculosis
      Malaria
    Anaphylaxis
    Neoplasms (especially leukemia, lymphoma, and car-
      cinoma of lung, prostate, or pancreas)
  Thrombotic thrombocytopenic purpura
  Idiopathic thrombocytopenic purpura
  Posttransfusion purpura
  Wiskott-Aldrich syndrome
Thrombocytosis
Functional platelet disorders (e.g., thrombasthenia)
Coagulopathy (including drug-induced)

Vascular Causes
Vasculitis, small-vessel (hypersensitivity)
  Henoch-Schönlein purpura
  Rheumatoid arthritis
  Lupus erythematosus
  Cryoglobulinemia
  Sjögren's syndrome
  Waldenström's macroglobulinemia
  Lymphoproliferative disorders (especially Hodgkin's
    disease, lymphosarcoma)
  Hyperglobulinemic purpura
Wegener's granulomatosis
Hereditary hemorrhagic telangiectasia

Pseudoxanthoma elasticum
Capillary fragility syndromes

Extravascular Causes
Aging
Trauma
Steroids
Amyloidosis
Ehlers-Danlos syndrome
Scurvy

Reference
1. General reference 22.

10-F. Pruritus

Dermatologic Disorders
Scabies
Ringworm
Dermatitis herpetiformis
Atopic dermatitis
Miliaria
Insect bites
Pediculosis
Contact dermatitis
Psoriasis
Lichen planus
Urticaria

Pruritus without Diagnostic Skin Lesions
Psychogenic states
Dry skin
Senile pruritus
Drug sensitivity or addiction (especially opiates, amphetamines)
Chronic renal failure with secondary hyperparathyroidism
Obstructive liver disease
   Biliary cirrhosis
   Bile duct obstruction, extrahepatic

Cholestasis, drug-induced (oral contraceptives,
    phenothiazines, chlorpropamide)
  Intrahepatic cholestasis of pregnancy
Lymphoma (rarely other neoplasms)
Polycythemia vera
Hyperthyroidism
Carcinoid tumor
Infestation (including scabies, lice, parasites)

Reference
1. Fitzpatrick TB: Fundamentals of Dermatologic
   Diagnosis. In general reference 22, p 10.

10-G. Generalized Pustules

Acne vulgaris
Pyogenic infection, especially:
  Disseminated staphylococcal
  Disseminated gonococcal
  Bacterial endocarditis
Viral infection (especially vaccinia, variola)
Syphilis, secondary
Mycobacterial or fungal infection (occasionally)
Pustular psoriasis
Drugs, especially:
  Sulfonamides
  Phenytoin
  Iodides
  Bromides

Reference
1. General reference 22.

10-H. Telangiectasia

Normal variant
Wind and/or sun exposure
Pregnancy or estrogen therapy
Chronic liver disease (especially cirrhosis)
Topical steroid therapy (long-term)
Systemic lupus erythematosus
Dermatomyositis
Systemic sclerosis, CRST syndrome
Osler-Rendu-Weber syndrome (hereditary hemorrhagic
  telangiectasia)
Ataxia telangiectasia
Fabry's disease
States associated with prolonged vasodilatation (e.g.,
  varicose veins, rosacea, polycythemia vera)
Radiation dermatitis
Urticaria pigmentosa
Carcinoid tumor, metastatic
Xeroderma pigmentosum
Poikiloderma
Generalized essential telangiectasia

Reference
1. General reference 22.

10-I. Urticaria

Atopic conditions
Specific antigen sensitivity (e.g., foods, Hymenoptera
    venom, helminths)
Physical agents
    Pressure, mechanical irritation
    Cold
    Heat
    Light
Drugs
    Opiates
    Antibiotics (especially penicillin, sulfonamides)
    Curare
    X-ray contrast media
    Aspirin, nonsteroidal anti-inflammatory agents
    Azo dyes
Transfusion of blood or blood products
Cryoglobulins, cryoproteins
Serum sickness
Hepatitis B, acute
Lupus erythematosus
Necrotizing vasculitis
Mastocytosis (urticaria pigmentosa)
Occult malignancy
Idiopathic

Reference
1. General reference 22.

10-J. Generalized Vesicles and Bullae

Physical agents
  Radiation
  Burns
  Chemicals
  Mechanical irritation, trauma
Drugs
  Barbiturates
  Penicillins
  Sulfonamides
  Phenytoin
  Phenylbutazone
  Allopurinol
  Halides
  Phenolphthalein
  Nalidixic acid
Allergic contact dermatitis (e.g., poison ivy)
Viral infection
  Varicella
  Cowpox, vaccinia
  Variola (smallpox)
  Herpes simplex
  Herpes zoster
  Enterovirus (ECHO, coxsackievirus)
  Adenovirus
Bacterial infection, pyogenic
  Disseminated gonococcus, *Pseudomonas*
  Impetigo, erysipelas
  Toxic epidermal necrolysis
Syphilis, congenital
Rickettsialpox
Erythema multiforme bullosum, Stevens-Johnson syndrome
Pemphigus
Pemphigoid
Dermatitis herpetiformis
Behçet's disease
Porphyria (all types except acute intermittent porphyria)
Lupus erythematosus

Reference
1. General reference 22.

11
Musculoskeletal System

11-A. Shoulder Pain

Fracture
Contusion
Acromial-clavicular joint separation
Rotator cuff injury
Bursitis
Bicipital tendonitis (long head)
Referred pain
   Diaphragmatic irritation
      Blood or gas in peritoneal or pleural cavity
      Subphrenic abscess
      Neoplasm
      Lower-lobe pleuropulmonary inflammatory disease
   Apical lung cancer (Pancoast syndrome)
   Cervical radiculopathy
   Angina pectoris and/or myocardial infarction
Osteoarthritis
Infectious arthritis
Rheumatoid arthritis
Crystalline arthritis
Arthritis associated with collagen-vascular disease
Shoulder-hand syndrome
Neoplasm, primary or metastatic
Local arterial, venous, or lymphatic occlusion
Thoracic outlet syndromes

Cervical and first-rib syndromes, scalenus anterior
    syndrome
Hyperabduction syndrome
Costoclavicular syndrome
Myalgias and arthralgias
Fibrositis syndromes
Psychogenic pain

References
1. Jacobs RC: Painful Shoulder. In general reference 4,
    p 261.
2. Rodnan GP (Ed): *Primer on the Rheumatic Diseases*
    (7th ed). *JAMA* 224(5) suppl: 86, 1973.

11-B. Back Pain

Functional, mechanical causes: Postural imbalance
    Anteroposterior (e.g., pregnancy)
    Lateral (e.g., scoliosis, unequal leg lengths)
Trauma
    Lumbar strain or sprain
    Lumbosacral disk herniation
    Vertebral fracture (compression or other)
    Subluxation of facet joints
Osteoarthritis, spondylosis
Rheumatoid arthritis
Spondylitis and/or sacroiliitis
    Ankylosing spondylitis
    Colitic (enteropathic) spondylitis
    Psoriatic arthritis
    Behçet's syndrome
    Reiter's syndrome
    Familial Mediterranean fever
    Syphilis
    Ochronosis
Spinal stenosis
    Congenital
    Degenerative
    Postsurgical

Posttraumatic
Paget's disease
Fluorosis
Spinal or vertebral tumor
  Benign (e.g., hemangioma, meningioma, osteoid osteoma)
  Malignant
    Primary (e.g., multiple myeloma, ependymoma, osteogenic sarcoma)
    Metastatic, especially:
      Prostate
      Breast
      Lung
      Kidney
      Thyroid
      Gastrointestinal tract
Infection (e.g., disk space infection, vertebral osteomyelitis)
  Bacteria (usually secondary to hematogenous spread)
  Brucella
  Mycobacteria
  Fungi
Congenital causes
  Facet tropism
  Transitional vertebrae
  Spina bifida
  Spondylolysis, spondylolisthesis
Hyperparathyroidism
Osteomalacia (e.g., vitamin D–resistant rickets)
Scheuermann's disease (epiphysitis)
Radium poisoning
Osteogenesis imperfecta
Referred pain
  Vascular disease (especially abdominal aortic aneurysm, Leriche syndrome)
  Hip pain
  Pelvic or prostatic inflammation or tumor
  Retroperitoneal hematoma or tumor
  Renal disease, e.g.:
    Stone
    Infection
    Tumor
    Polycystic kidney disease
  Abdominal disease (e.g., intestinal, pancreatic)
Psychoneurotic causes
  Hysteria
  Malingering

References
1. Mankin HJ, Adams RD: Pain in the Back and Neck. In general reference 1, p 38.
2. Levine DB: The Painful Low Back. In general reference 23, p 1044.
3. Keim HA, Kirkaldy-Willis WH: Low Back Pain. *Clin Symp* 32(6), 1980.

11-C. Myalgias

Fibrositis
Connective-tissue disease
   Polymyalgia rheumatica
   Rheumatoid arthritis
   Polymyositis, dermatomyositis
   Lupus erythematosus
   Polyarteritis nodosa
   Scleroderma
Systemic infection, especially:
   Viral illness, e.g.:
      Influenza
      Coxsackievirus infection
      Arbovirus infection
      Hepatitis
      Rabies
      Poliomyelitis
   Rheumatic fever
   Salmonellosis
   Tularemia
   Brucellosis
   Glanders
   Trichinosis
   Leptospirosis
   Relapsing fever
   Malaria
Rhabdomyolysis (see 11-D)
Drugs (e.g., amphotericin B, clofibrate, carbenoxolone)
Hypothyroidism
Hyperparathyroidism

Hypoglycemic myopathy
Congenital enzyme deficiency (e.g., phosphorylase
    [McArdle's disease], phosphofructokinase)
Polyneuropathy (e.g., Guillain-Barré disease)
Ischemic atherosclerotic disease (i.e., intermittent
    claudication)

Reference
1. Section 14: Diseases of Striated Muscle. In general reference 1, p 2040.

11-D. Muscle Weakness

Acute or Subacute*
Electrolyte abnormality
    Hyperkalemia
    Hypokalemia
    Hypercalcemia
    Hypermagnesemia
    Hypophosphatemia
Rhabdomyolysis
    Extreme muscular exertion
    Prolonged seizures
    Hyperthermia
    Extensive crush injury or muscle infarction
    Influenza
    Hypokalemia
    Hypophosphatemia
    Alcoholic myopathy
    Meyer-Betz paroxysmal myoglobinuria
    Haff disease
    McArdle's disease
Polymyositis, dermatomyositis
Infection, especially:
    Viral, e.g.:
        Influenza

---

*Developing over days to weeks. See also "Intermittent and/or Transient" following.

          Coxsackievirus infection
          Rabies
          Poliomyelitis
      Trichinosis
      Toxoplasmosis
      Botulism
Peripheral neuropathy, acute (see 12-R)
Thyrotoxicosis
Corticosteroid therapy
Organophosphorus poisoning

Chronic†
Muscular dystrophy, especially:
    Duchenne's
    Facioscapulohumeral
    Limb-girdle
    Myotonic
Endocrine disorders
    Hyperthyroidism or hypothyroidism
    Hyperparathyroidism
    Vitamin D deficiency (e.g., vitamin D–deficiency rickets)
    Corticosteroid therapy
    Cushing's syndrome
    Acromegaly
Connective-tissue disease
    Lupus erythematosus
    Rheumatoid arthritis
    Polymyositis, dermatomyositis
    Sjögren's syndrome
    Mixed connective-tissue disease
Alcoholic myopathy
Chronic polymyopathy, e.g.:
    Glycogen storage disease
    Central core disease
    McArdle's disease
    Familial periodic paralysis with progressive myopathy
Progressive neural-muscular atrophy, e.g.:
    Amyotrophic lateral sclerosis
    Multiple sclerosis
    Werdnig-Hoffmann disease
    Peroneal muscular atrophy (Charcot-Marie-Tooth
      disease)
    Chronic peripheral neuropathy (e.g., arsenic, lead, nu-
      tritional) (see also 12-R)

Intermittent and/or Transient
Electrolyte abnormality
    Hypokalemia
    Hyperkalemia

Hypophosphatemia
Hypercalcemia
Hypermagnesemia
Hyperkalemic or hypokalemic periodic paralysis
Aminoglycosides, especially:
  Neomycin
  Streptomycin
  Kanamycin
  Polymyxin B
Myasthenia gravis
Eaton-Lambert syndrome
Acute thyrotoxic myopathy
Thyrotoxic periodic paralysis
Paramyotonia congenita
Adynamia episodica hereditaria

Reference
1. Section 14: Diseases of Striated Muscle. In general reference 1, p 2040.

†Developing over months.

11-E. Polyarticular Arthritis

Rheumatoid arthritis*
Juvenile rheumatoid arthritis*
Rheumatic fever*
Ankylosing spondylitis*
Collagen-vascular diseases
  Lupus erythematosus*
  Scleroderma*
  Polymyositis, dermatomyositis*
  Mixed connective-tissue disease
  Polyarteritis nodosa* (rare)
  Henoch-Schönlein purpura* (rare)
  Wegener's granulomatosis* (rare)
  Other vasculitides* (e.g., allergic granulomatosis) (rare)
  Polymyalgia rheumatica*
Immunologically mediated diseases
  Serum sickness*

Hyperglobulinemic purpura*
Hypogammaglobulinemia*
Mixed cryoglobulinemia* (rare)
Systemic diseases
  Sjögren's syndrome*
  Reiter's syndrome*
  Psoriasis*
  Behçet's syndrome*
  Inflammatory bowel disease*
    Ulcerative colitis
    Regional enteritis
  Pancreatic disease
    Carcinoma
    Pancreatitis
  Whipple's disease*
  Familial Mediterranean fever*
  Amyloidosis
  Sarcoidosis*
  Hematologic disorders
    Leukemia*
    Lymphoma*
    Multiple myeloma*
    Hemophilia
    Hemoglobinopathies* (especially sickle cell anemia,
      thalassemia)
  Storage diseases* (e.g., Gaucher's disease, Fabry's
    disease, hyperlipoproteinemia)
  Ochronosis
  Hemochromatosis
  Wilson's disease
  Acromegaly
  Hypothyroidism
Degenerative joint disease
Trauma
Neuropathic arthropathy (e.g., tabes dorsalis, diabetes
  mellitus, syringomyelia)
Joint tumor
  Pigmented villonodular synovitis
  Hemangioma
  Sarcoma
Infection*
  Bacterial (especially gonococcus, staphylococcus,
    pneumococcus)
  Viral (especially hepatitis B, mumps, rubella)
  Tuberculous
  Fungal
  Rickettsial
  Parasitic

Others
   Gout*
   Pseudogout*
   Hypertrophic osteoarthropathy
   Intermittent hydrarthrosis*
   Palindromic rheumatism*
   Radiation
   Relapsing polychondritis*
   Acute tropical polyarthritis*
Nonarticular rheumatism
   Bursitis*
   Periarthritis*
   Tendinitis*
   Tenosynovitis*
   Epicondylitis
   Myositis
   Fibrositis
   Fasciitis

Reference
1. General reference 23.

*Usually inflammatory (i.e., joints painful, swollen, stiff, often erythematous and warm).

11-F. Monoarticular (or Oligoarticular) Arthritis

Juvenile rheumatoid arthritis
Ankylosing spondylitis
Rheumatoid arthritis (rare)
Systemic diseases
   Psoriasis
   Behçet's syndrome
   Inflammatory bowel disease (ulcerative colitis, regional enteritis)
   Pancreatic disease (carcinoma, pancreatitis)
   Whipple's disease
   Familial Mediterranean fever
   Hematologic disorders

Leukemia
Lymphoma
Hemophilia
Hemoglobinopathies (especially sickle cell anemia,
thalassemia)
Storage diseases (e.g., Gaucher's, Fabry's)
Acromegaly
Degenerative joint disease
Trauma
Neuropathic arthropathy (e.g., tabes dorsalis, diabetes
mellitus, syringomyelia)
Joint tumors (e.g., pigmented villonodular synovitis,
hemangioma, sarcoma)
Infection
Bacterial (especially gonococcus, staphylococcus,
pneumococcus)
Viral (especially hepatitis B, rubella, mumps)
Tuberculous
Fungal
Rickettsial
Parasitic
Others
Gout
Pseudogout
Intermittent hydrarthrosis
Palindromic rheumatism
Radiation
Relapsing polychondritis
Nonarticular rheumatism
Bursitis
Periarthritis
Tendinitis
Tenosynovitis
Epicondylitis
Myositis
Fibrositis
Fasciitis

Reference
1. General reference 23.

11-G. Characteristics of Synovial Fluid

	Normal	Noninflammatory	Inflammatory	Purulent	Hemorrhagic
Color	Clear to pale yellow	Xanthochromic	Xantho-chromic to white	White	
Clarity	Transparent	Transparent	Translucent to opaque	Opaque	
Viscosity	High	High	Low	Low*	
Mucin clot	Good	Good to fair	Fair to poor	Poor	
Spontaneous clot	None	Often	Often	Often	
WBCs/mm³	< 150	< 3,000	3,000–50,000	> 50,000	
% Polymorphs	< 25	< 25	> 70	> 90	
Conditions in which findings are likely to occur		Osteoarthritis Trauma Aseptic necrosis Lupus erythematosus	Rheumatoid arthritis Reiter's syndrome Psoriatic arthritis	Bacterial or tuberculous arthritis	Trauma Anticoagulation Neuropathic arthropathy: Charcot joints Joint tumor

Normal	Noninflammatory	Inflammatory	Purulent	Hemorrhagic
	Polyarteritis nodosa Amyloidosis	Inflammatory bowel disease arthritis Viral arthritis Rheumatic fever Acute gout or pseudogout		Hematologic disorders (especially hemophilia, sickle cell trait or disease)

Source: Group designations from Ropes MW, Bauer W: *Synovial Fluid Changes in Joint Diseases.* Cambridge, Mass.: Harvard University Press, 1953. Table modified from McCarty DJ: Synovial Fluid. In McCarty DJ (Ed): *Arthritis and Allied Conditions* (9th ed), Philadelphia: Lea & Febiger, 1979, pp 52–56. Copyright © 1979 by Lea & Febiger.
*May be high in infection with coagulase-positive staphylococcus.

11-H. Clubbing

Usually with Hypertrophic Osteoarthropathy
Neoplasm
  Intrathoracic
    Lung
    Pleura
    Mediastinum (Hodgkin's disease)
    Thymus
  Esophagus, stomach
  Intestine
  Liver
Other pulmonary disorders
  Lung abscess
  Empyema
  Chronic pneumonitis
  Pneumoconiosis
  Bronchiectasis
  Tuberculosis
  Cystic fibrosis
Idiopathic, hereditary (pachydermoperiostitis)

Usually without Hypertrophic Osteoarthropathy
Genetic
Subacute bacterial endocarditis
Cyanotic congenital heart disease
Chronic liver disease (e.g., biliary cirrhosis)
Intestinal disorders
  Ulcerative colitis
  Regional enteritis
  Sprue, steatorrhea
  Bacterial or amebic dysentery
  Tuberculosis, intestinal
Hyperparathyroidism
Graves' disease (thyroid acropachy)
Occupational trauma (e.g., jackhammer operation)

Unilateral
Aneurysm of aorta or of subclavian, innominate, or
    brachial artery
Shoulder subluxation
Hemiplegia
Axillary or apical lung tumor

Unidigital
Median nerve injury
Sarcoidosis
Tophaceous gout

Reference
1. Howell DS: Hypertrophic Osteoarthropathy. In general reference 23, p 977.

11-I. Raynaud's Phenomenon

Raynaud's disease
Chronic arterial disease
   Atherosclerosis
   Thromboangiitis obliterans
   Thrombosis
   Embolism
Collagen-vascular disease
   Scleroderma
   Lupus erythematosus
   Rheumatoid arthritis
   Polyarteritis nodosa
   Mixed connective-tissue disease
   Polymyositis, dermatomyositis
   Sjögren's syndrome
Occupational exposure
   Vibration (e.g., pneumatic tools)
   Percussion (e.g., typing)
   Vinyl chloride polymerization
Drugs, toxins
   Heavy metals (lead, arsenic, thallium)
   Methysergide, ergot compounds
   Propranolol
Hematologic disorders
   Dysproteinemias (e.g., multiple myeloma, Waldenström's macroglobulinemia)
   Polycythemia vera
   Leukemia
   Cryoglobulinemia
   Cold agglutinin phenomenon

Neurologic disorders
   Peripheral neuropathy
   Hemiplegia
   Intervertebral disk herniation
   Spinal cord tumor
   Multiple sclerosis
   Transverse myelitis
   Syringomyelia
Carpal tunnel syndrome
Thoracic outlet syndrome
Posttraumatic reflex sympathetic dystrophy
Post-cold injury (e.g., frostbite)
Acromegaly
Myxedema
Fabry's disease

References

1. General reference 1.
2. Spittell JA: Raynaud's Phenomenon and Allied Vaso-spastic Conditions. In Fairbairn JF, Juergens JL, Spittell JA (Eds): *Allen-Barker-Hines Peripheral Vascular Diseases* (4th ed). Philadelphia: Saunders, 1972, p 387.

11-J. Osteomalacia

Vitamin D deficiency
   Dietary deficiency
   Insufficient sun exposure
   Malabsorption (e.g., pancreatic insufficiency, small-intestine disease, postgastrectomy)
Disordered vitamin D metabolism
   Chronic renal failure
   Anticonvulsant therapy
   Chronic liver disease (e.g., biliary cirrhosis)
Chronic acidosis (e.g., distal renal tubular acidosis, ureterosigmoidostomy)
Phosphate depletion (see 1-0)
Impaired renal tubular phosphate reabsorption
   Vitamin D–resistant rickets

    Fanconi syndrome (hereditary or acquired)
    Tumor phosphaturia
    Neurofibromatosis
    Neonatal (transient)
Miscellaneous
    Osteopetrosis
    Hypophosphatasia
    Fluorosis

References

1. Dent CE, Stamp TCB: Vitamin D, Rickets, and Osteomalacia. In Avioli LV, Krane SM (Eds): *Metabolic Bone Disease.* New York: Academic, 1977, p 237.
2. Krane SM, Holick MF: Metabolic Bone Disease. In general reference 1, p 1849.

11-K. Osteopenia*

Aging (especially postmenopause)†
Immobilization†
Nutritional causes
    Calcium and/or vitamin D deficiency
    Malnutrition, malabsorption
    Postgastrectomy
    Scurvy
Corticosteroid excess†
    Cushing's syndrome or disease
    Steroid therapy
Other endocrine disorders
    Hypogonadism (e.g., Klinefelter's syndrome, Turner's
        syndrome)†
    Thyrotoxicosis
    Acromegaly
    Hyperparathyroidism
    Hypopituitarism
    Diabetes mellitus
Inherited connective-tissue diseases
    Homocystinuria
    Marfan's syndrome

 Ehlers-Danlos syndrome
 Osteogenesis imperfecta
Rheumatoid arthritis†
Ankylosing spondylitis
Malignancy, especially:
 Lymphoma
 Leukemia
 Multiple myeloma
 Waldenström's macroglobulinemia
 Systemic mastocytosis
Heparin therapy (chronic)†
Chronic obstructive pulmonary disease†
Chronic acidosis (especially renal tubular acidosis,
 metabolic acidosis secondary to high-protein diet)
Alcoholism
Hepatic insufficiency, cirrhosis (alcoholic or other)
Methotrexate†
Epilepsy
Chronic renal failure (renal osteodystrophy)
Paget's disease (with predominantly lytic lesions)
Juvenile (idiopathic)†
Cystic fibrosis†
Riley-Day syndrome
Menkes' syndrome
Down's syndrome
Hypophosphatasia, adult variety

References

1. Avioli LV: Osteoporosis: Pathogenesis and Therapy. In
 Avioli LV, Krane SM (Eds): *Metabolic Bone Disease.*
 New York: Academic, 1977, p 307.
2. Thomsen DL, Frame B: Involutional Osteopenia: Current Concepts. *Ann Intern Med* 85:789, 1976.

*Decreased bone mass.
†Characterized on bone biopsy by decreased bone mass with normal mineral-to-matrix ratio.

11-L. Antinuclear Antibodies

Disease	Antibodies Most Commonly Associated
Systemic lupus erythematosus	Antinative (double-stranded) DNA
	Anti-DNA protein
	Anti-single-stranded DNA
	Antinuclear ribonucleoprotein
	Anti-Sm
	Antihistones (especially with drug-induced lupus)
Progressive systemic sclerosis	Antinucleolar
Polymyositis, dermatomyositis	Anti-PM-I
	Anti-Mi
Mixed connective-tissue disease	Anti-extractable nuclear antigen (ENA)
Sjögren's syndrome	Anti-SS-A, SS-B
	Anti-Ro
Rheumatoid arthritis	Anti-single-stranded DNA

Reference
1. Reichlin M: Introduction to Systemic Rheumatic Diseases: Nosology and Overlap Syndromes. In general reference 23, p 687.

11-M. Rheumatoid Factor

Aging
Rheumatoid arthritis
Lupus erythematosus
Scleroderma
Dermatomyositis, polymyositis
Infections
   Syphilis
   Subacute bacterial endocarditis
   Infectious mononucleosis
   Viral hepatitis
   Tuberculosis
   Leprosy
   Parasitic infection (e.g., schistosomiasis)
   Following extensive immunizations
Sjögren's syndrome
Chronic active hepatitis
Lymphoma
Waldenström's macroglobulinemia
Mixed cryoglobulinemia
Hyperglobulinemic purpura
Chronic lung disease
   Pneumoconioses (e.g., silicosis, asbestosis)
   Sarcoidosis
   Interstitial fibrosis, idiopathic
Multiple transfusions
Renal transplantation

Reference

1. Gilliland BC, Mannik M: Rheumatoid Arthritis. In general reference 1, p 1872.

11-N. Lupus Erythematosus Criteria*

Facial erythema (butterfly rash)
Discoid lupus erythematosus
Raynaud's phenomenon
Alopecia
Photosensitivity
Oral or nasopharyngeal ulceration
Arthritis without deformity
LE cells or positive ANA
Chronic false-positive serologic test for syphilis
Proteinuria > 3.5 gm/day
Cellular casts in urine (red cell, hemoglobin, granular,
    tubular, or mixed)
Pleuritis and/or pericarditis
Psychosis and/or convulsions
One or more of the following: hemolytic anemia,
    leukopenia (WBC count < 4,000/mm³), throm-
    bocytopenia (platelet count < 100,000/mm³)

*From Cohen AS, Reynolds WE, Franklin EC, et al: Preliminary Criteria for the Classification of Systemic Lupus Erythematosus. *Bull Rheum Dis* 21:643, 1971. Diagnosis of systemic lupus can be made if four or more of the above criteria are present, serially or simultaneously, during any period of observation.

12
Nervous System

12-A. Dizziness and Vertigo

Dizziness
Hyperventilation
Anxiety, psychosomatic causes
Hypoxia
Anemia
Orthostatic hypotension

True Vertigo
Seizure aura
Oculomotor disorders (e.g., diplopia)
Lesions of cerebellum, cerebral cortex, cervical muscles
 (rare)
Vestibular system lesions
 Ménière's disease
 Benign positional vertigo of Bárány
 Vestibular neuronitis, acute labyrinthitis
 Purulent labyrinthitis associated with meningitis
 Serous labyrinthitis associated with middle ear infec-
  tion
 Drugs
  Alcohol
  Quinine
  Streptomycin, gentamicin (aminoglycoside anti-
   biotics)
  Salicylates

Trauma/hemorrhage into middle ear
Cogan's syndrome
Vestibular nerve compression
    Tumor (especially acoustic neuroma)
    Meningeal inflammation
    Vascular compression
Brain stem lesion
    Transient ischemic attack or infarction involving ver-
        tebral or basilar arteries
    Multiple sclerosis
Vertebrobasilar migraine

Reference

1. General reference 24, p 178.

12-B. Headache

Tension
Ocular causes, especially:
    Astigmatism
    Hypermetropia
    Glaucoma
    Iridocyclitis
Disease of teeth or gums
Disease of ligaments, muscles, joints or upper spine
Sinus infection or blockage
Vasomotor rhinitis
Hypertension, hypotension
Hypercapnia
Febrile illness
Drugs (especially theophylline, indomethacin, nitro-
    glycerin)
Temporal arteritis
Following lumbar puncture
Migraine headache
    Typical
    Atypical
    Basilar artery type
Cluster headache
Following head trauma

Evolving atherosclerotic thrombosis (especially of internal
    carotid artery, anterior or middle cerebral artery,
    basilar artery)
Subdural hematoma
Intracranial berry aneurysm
Intracranial angioma
Intracranial hemorrhage
Meningitis, encephalitis, brain abscess
Brain tumor

Reference
1. General reference 24, p 95.

12-C. Paresthesias

Peripheral neuropathy (see 12-R)
Peripheral nerve entrapment, compression, or trauma
    (e.g., intervertebral disk herniation, thoracic outlet
    syndrome, carpal tunnel syndrome)
Arteriosclerotic peripheral vascular disease
Spinal cord disease
  Spinal cord or nerve root compression
  Tabes dorsalis
  Subacute combined degeneration of spinal cord
  Strachan's syndrome
Metabolic imbalance
  Hypocalcemia
  Respiratory alkalosis

Reference
1. General reference 1.

12-D. Syncope

Neurological and/or Mechanical Causes
Mediated by vagal stimulation and/or autonomic insufficiency
  Vasovagal reaction
  Carotid sinus syncope
  Micturition syncope
  Glossopharyngeal neuralgia
  Orthostatic hypotension
  Prolonged recumbency or inactivity
  Peripheral neuropathy with autonomic fiber involvement (e.g., diabetes, tabes dorsalis)
  Drugs (e.g., nitrates, antihypertensives, ganglionic blockers, alcohol)
  Sympathectomy
  Primary autonomic insufficiency
Seizure
Head trauma
Reduced venous return to the heart
  Hypovolemia
  Valsalva maneuver (including cough)
  Atrial myxoma or thrombus

Cardiopulmonary Causes
Cardiac arrhythmias (bradyarrhythmias, tachyarrhythmias, atrioventricular block) (see 2-O)
Pulmonary embolism
Myocardial infarction with cardiogenic shock
Pericardial tamponade
Aortic stenosis
Idiopathic hypertrophic subaortic stenosis
Pulmonic stenosis
Primary pulmonary hypertension
Other causes of hypotension

Cerebrovascular Causes
Atherosclerotic disease of carotid and/or cerebral vessels (especially vertebral-basilar insufficiency)
Takayasu's disease
Hypertensive encephalopathy

Metabolic Causes
Anemia
Hypoxia
Respiratory alkalosis
Hypoglycemia

Psychological Causes
Anxiety, hysteria

Reference
1. General reference 24, p 231.

12-E. Tinnitus*

"Physiologic"
Inner ear disease (usually associated with sensorineural
    hearing loss)
Middle ear disease (usually associated with conductive
    hearing loss)
Bruit of neck vessel, intracranial arteriovenous malforma-
    tion

Reference
1. General reference 24, p 178.

*See also 12-F.

12-F. Deafness

Sensorineural (Inner Ear)
Aging
Prolonged exposure to loud noise
Drugs
    Salicylates
    Quinine
    Aminoglycoside antibiotics
    Furosemide, ethacrynic acid

Meningitis
Chronic middle or inner ear infection
Mumps
Syphilis
Ménière's disease
Tumor of eighth nerve or cerebellopontine angle (especially acoustic neuroma, cholesteatoma)
Multiple sclerosis
Eighth nerve infarction
Hereditary or congenital causes (e.g., congenital rubella)

Conductive (Middle Ear)
Cerumen impaction
Otosclerosis
Otitis media
Perforated tympanic membrane
Trauma (including temporal bone fracture, bleeding into middle ear)
Mucopolysaccharidoses

Reference
1. General reference 24, p 178

12-G. Ataxia

Cerebellar Disease (Cerebellar Ataxia)
Alcoholic cerebellar degeneration, Wernicke's disease
Multiple sclerosis
Tumor
Vascular occlusion (basilar artery or its branches)
Encephalitis (e.g., subacute sclerosing panencephalitis)
Brain abscess
Cranial trauma
Following hyperthermia
Hypoxic encephalopathy
Nonwilsonian hepatocerebral degeneration (post–hepatic coma)
Hypoparathyroidism

Congenital
Hereditary (e.g., phenylketonuria, Hartnup disease, lipid
      storage diseases, ataxia telangiectasia)

Loss of Postural or Proprioceptive Sense
(Sensory Ataxia)
Polyneuropathy
Tabes dorsalis
Syphilitic meningomyelitis
Multiple sclerosis
Subacute combined degeneration of the spinal cord
Spinal cord tumor
Hereditary (e.g., Friedreich's ataxia)

Others
Myxedema
Frontal lobe disease (e.g., senile dementia)

Reference
1. General references 1 and 24.

12-H. Acute Confusional State*

Delirium†
Drug withdrawal after chronic intoxication, especially:
      Alcohol
      Barbiturates
      Other sedatives
Drug intoxication, especially:
      Atropine
      Amphetamines
      Bromides
      Caffeine
      Camphor
      Ergot
      Scopolamine
Infectious and febrile illness, especially:
      Septicemia

---

*See also 12-I and 12-N.
†An acute, transient confusional state characterized by mental
alertness, gross disorientation, hallucinations, psychomotor and
autonomic hyperactivity.

Pneumonia
Typhoid fever
Rheumatic fever
Central nervous system disorders
Cerebrovascular disease (especially involving temporal lobes or upper brain stem)
Brain tumor
Encephalitis (especially viral)
Meningitis
Head trauma (e.g., subdural hematoma)
Following seizures
Thyrotoxicosis
Steroid psychosis (rare)

Other Acute Confusional States‡

Metabolic causes
Electrolyte disorders, especially:
Hyponatremia
Hypercalcemia
Hypokalemia
Hypoxia
Hypercarbia
Hypoglycemia
Hepatic encephalopathy
Uremia
Wernicke's disease
Porphyria
Drug intoxication, e.g.:
Barbiturates
Narcotics
Bromides
Central nervous system disease
Cerebrovascular disease (see 12-O)
Brain tumor
Brain abscess
Meningitis
Encephalitis
Subdural hematoma, epidural hematoma
Febrile illness
Acute psychosis (e.g., postoperative, postpartum)
Preexisting dementia with superimposed stress (e.g., serious illness) (see 12-I)

Reference

1 General reference 24, p 259.

‡Confusional states not associated with psychomotor or autonomic hyperactivity.

12-I. Dementia*

Senile dementia, Alzheimer's disease
Cerebral arteriosclerosis, multiple cerebrovascular accidents
Pick's disease (circumscribed cerebral atrophy)
Parkinson's disease
Korsakoff's psychosis
Brain tumor
Head trauma (e.g., contusion, hemorrhage, subdural hematoma)
Brain abscess
Chronic meningoencephalitis (e.g., cryptococcosis, paretic neurosyphilis)
Hypoxic encephalopathy
Bromism
Chronic barbiturate intoxication
Myoclonic epilepsy
Normal-pressure hydrocephalus
Hepatocerebral degeneration (acquired, post-hepatic coma)
Dialysis dementia
Pernicious anemia, subacute combined degeneration of spinal cord
Pellagra
Myxedema
Cushing's disease
Creutzfeldt-Jakob disease
Schilder's disease (diffuse cerebral sclerosis)
Hereditary diseases
   Huntington's chorea
   Wilson's disease
   Lipid storage diseases (e.g., Tay-Sachs, leukodystrophies)
   Mucopolysaccharidoses

Reference
1. General reference 24, p 270.

*Deterioration of intellectual and cognitive function without clouding of consciousness or disturbances in perception. See also 12-H and 12-N.

12-J. Tremor

Static (present at rest, decreased with movement)
  Parkinson's disease
  Postencephalitic parkinsonism
  Wilson's disease
  Phenothiazines (tardive dyskinesia)
  Brain tumor
Action (present with movement, decreased at rest)
  Anxiety
  Intense muscular fatigue
  Senile and/or familial (benign essential)
  Alcohol withdrawal
  Meningoencephalitis (e.g., viral; paretic neurosyphilis)
  Hyperthyroidism
  Pheochromocytoma
  Carcinoid syndrome
  Steroids
  Lithium
Rest and intention (present at rest, worse with movement)
  Multiple sclerosis
  Peripheral neuropathy
  Parkinson's disease
  Cerebellar degeneration
  Wilson's disease
  Hysteria
  Drugs (e.g., theophylline, caffeine, epinephrine, ter-
    butaline)
Ataxic (increased at terminal phase of voluntary move-
  ment) (see 12-G).

References

1. Adams RD: Tremor, Chorea, Athetosis, Ataxia, and Other Abnormalities of Movement and Posture. In general reference 1, p 90.
2. Jankovic J, Fahn S: Physiologic and Pathologic Tremors: Diagnosis, Mechanism, and Management. *Ann Intern Med* 93:460–465, 1980.

12-K. Choreoathetosis

Hereditary diseases, especially:
  Wilson's disease
  Huntington's chorea
  Lesch-Nyhan disease
  Lipid storage disease (e.g., Niemann-Pick)
  Familial paroxysmal choreoathetosis
  Dystonia musculorum deformans
Drugs (especially phenothiazines, haloperidol, L-dopa)
Rheumatic fever (Sydenham's chorea)
Pregnancy
Hyperthyroidism
Kernicterus
Perinatal hypoxia or injury
Hypoxic encephalopathy
Nonwilsonian hepatocerebral degeneration (post–hepatic
  coma)
Lupus erythematosus
Polycythemia vera
Senile chorea
Thalamic infarct or hemorrhage (unilateral choreo-
  athetosis)
Posthemiplegic states (unilateral choreoathetosis)

References
1. General reference 24.
2. Adams RD: Tremor, Chorea, Athetosis, Ataxia, and
   Other Abnormalities of Movement and Posture. In general reference 1, p 90.

12-L. Nystagmus

Pendular*
Congenital
Spasmus nutans
Associated with bilateral central loss of vision before two
   years of age
   Albinism
   Aniridia
   Bilateral chorioretinitis
   Congenital cataracts
   Corneal scarring
   Optic atrophy
Multiple sclerosis
Prolonged work in dim light (miner's nystagmus)

Jerk†
Horizontal
   Physiologic
      Attempt to fix on moving objects (opticokinetic nys-
         tagmus)
      Labyrinthine stimulation (e.g., cold water in auditory
         canal)
   Drugs (e.g., barbiturates, alcohol, phenytoin)
   Labyrinthine-vestibular disease (see 12-A)
   Encephalitis
   Cerebellar lesions (e.g., cerebellopontine angle tumor)
   Brain stem lesions (see "Vertical" below)
   Congenital
Vertical (usually associated with brain stem disease)
   Demyelinating disease (e.g., multiple sclerosis)
   Vascular disease involving brain stem (especially
      hypertensive infarction, posterior inferior cerebellar
      artery occlusion)
   Brain stem tumor
   Drugs (especially barbiturates, phenytoin)
   Cerebellar disease, especially of vermis (e.g., Wer-
      nicke's encephalopathy)
   Encephalitis
   Syringobulbia
   Meningioma, meningeal cyst

References
1. General reference 24, p 165.
2 General reference 11, p 447.

*Both components equal.
†Fast and slow components.

12-M. Seizures

Central Nervous System and Vascular Causes
Cerebrovascular disease (see 12-O)
  Thrombosis
  Embolism
  Hemorrhage (intracerebral or subarachnoid)
  Thrombophlebitis, vasculitis
  Infarction
  Arteriovenous malformation
Brain tumor (especially metastatic tumor, meningioma,
    astrocytoma)
Cerebral infection
  Encephalitis
  Meningitis (especially bacterial)
  Brain abscess
  Neurosyphilis
Head trauma
Hypoxic encephalopathy
Reduced cerebral blood flow (e.g., hypotension, Stokes-
    Adams syndrome, carotid sinus syncope)
Hypertensive encephalopathy
Toxemia of pregnancy
Alzheimer's disease (rare)

Metabolic Causes
Fever
Alcohol withdrawal
Barbiturate withdrawal
Drugs, toxins
  Amphetamines
  Phenothiazines
  Lidocaine
  Theophylline
  Penicillins
  Nalidixic acid
  Isoniazid
  Physostigmine and other anticholinergics
  Tricyclic antidepressants
  Vincristine
  Lithium
  Cycloserine
  Lead
  Arsenic
  Mercury
  Strychnine
  Camphor

Hypoglycemia
Hyperglycemia
Hyponatremia
Hypernatremia (or rapid correction of hypernatremia)
Hypocalcemia
Hypomagnesemia
Alkalosis, respiratory or metabolic
Uremia
Dialysis disequilibrium
Hepatic failure
Thyrotoxic storm
Pyridoxine deficiency

Congenital or Inherited Diseases
Congenital infection
   Toxoplasmosis
   Cytomegalovirus
   Syphilis
   Rubella (maternal)
Neonatal hypoxia or trauma
Lipid storage disease (e.g., Gaucher's disease)
Tuberous sclerosis
Sturge-Weber disease
Phenylketonuria
Argininosuccinic aciduria
Porphyria

Idiopathic

References
1. General reference 24, p 211.
2. Forster FM, Booker HE: The Epilepsies and Convulsive Disorders. In general reference 25, vol 2, chap 24, p 1.

12-N. Coma*

Drugs (especially anesthetics, sedatives, tranquilizers, aspirin)
Toxins (e.g., alcohol, methanol, carbon monoxide)
Hypoxia
Hypercapnia
Shock (e.g., septic, cardiogenic) (see 2-K)
Diabetic ketoacidosis, nonketotic hyperosmolar coma
Cerebrovascular accident (thrombosis, embolism, hemorrhage—see 12-O), especially involving upper brain stem
Hypertensive encephalopathy
Head trauma
Intracranial neoplasm
Seizures and postictal state
Meningitis, encephalitis, brain abscess
Hyperthermia or hypothermia
Hypernatremia or hyponatremia
Hypercalcemia
Hypoglycemia
Hepatic failure
Uremia
Myxedema
Thyroid storm
Adrenal insufficiency
Severe nutritional deficiency (especially of thiamine, niacin)
Hysteria

References

1. General reference 24, p 194.
2. Plum F, Posner JB: *Diagnosis of Stupor and Coma* (3rd ed). Philadelphia: Davis, 1980.

*See also 12-H and 12-I.

12-O. Cerebrovascular Disease

Thrombosis and/or Vascular Occlusion
Thrombosis
Vasculitis (mainly arteritis)
  Infectious
    Meningovascular syphilis
    Tuberculous meningitis
    Fungal meningitis
    Subacute bacterial meningitis
    Malaria
    Trichinosis
  Noninfectious
    Lupus erythematosus
    Polyarteritis nodosa
    Granulomatous arteritis
    Temporal arteritis
    Takayasu's disease
Hypertensive encephalopathy
Toxemia of pregnancy
Cerebral thrombophlebitis and/or venous sinus throm-
  bosis (usually associated with infection of ear, sinus,
  face, meninges)
Oral contraceptives
Sickle cell disease
Hyperproteinemia, hyperviscosity
Carotid artery trauma
Dissecting aneurysm or carotid artery (e.g., secondary to
  cystic medial necrosis or dissecting aortic aneurysm)
Migraine syndrome
Fibromuscular dysplasia
Moyamoya disease, multiple progressive intracranial arte-
  rial occlusions

Embolism
Atrial arrhythmias (especially atrial fibrillation—usually
  with atherosclerotic cardiovascular disease, rheu-
  matic valvular disease)
Rheumatic heart disease, especially mitral stenosis (with
  or without atrial fibrillation)
Myocardial infarction with mural thrombosis
Cardiac surgery
Prosthetic heart valve
Bacterial endocarditis with vegetations
Nonbacterial thrombotic endocardial vegetations (e.g.,
  associated with carcinomatosis)

Atherosclerotic embolism from other arteries
Aorta or carotid arteries (e.g., secondary to carotid
massage or arteriography)
Vertebral or basilar arteries
Pulmonary vein thrombosis (especially septic or tumor
emboli)
Fat embolism
Tumor embolism
Air embolism
Venous thromboembolism with cardiac or pulmonary
right-to-left shunt (paradoxic embolism)
Atrial myxoma
Trichinosis
Fabry's disease
Homocystinuria

Hemorrhage
Hypertension
Ruptured berry aneurysm
Ruptured arteriovenous malformation
Hemorrhagic disorders (e.g., thrombocytopenia, throm-
bocytosis, coagulopathy, disseminated intravascular
coagulation, anticoagulant therapy)
Cranial trauma
Hemorrhage into tumor
Hemorrhagic infarction
Ruptured mycotic aneurysm
Connective-tissue disease (especially lupus
erythematosus and polyarteritis nodosa)
Brain stem hemorrhage secondary to temporal lobe her-
niation

Reference
1. General reference 24, p 496.

12-P. Paralysis (or Paresis)*

Acute (Developing in Hours)
Spinal cord injury
Spinal cord hemorrhage (secondary to vascular malfor-
    mation, coagulopathy, anticoagulant therapy, trauma)
Spinal artery thrombosis, embolism, or occlusion
Dissecting aortic aneurysm
Aortic thrombosis
Acute necrotizing myelitis
Profound hypokalemia (serum K^+ < 2.5 mEq/L)†
Hyperkalemic or hypokalemic periodic paralysis†
Hypermagnesemia†

Subacute (Developing in Days)
Guillain-Barré syndrome
Viral myelitis (especially polio, rabies, herpes zoster)
Postinfectious myelitis (especially after measles,
    smallpox, chickenpox)
Postvaccinal myelitis (especially after rabies or smallpox
    vaccination)
Diphtheritic polyneuropathy
Botulism§
Subacute pyogenic meningomyelitis
Tuberculous meningomyelitis
Spinal cord or epidural abscess
Tumor with spinal cord compression
Acute demyelinating myelitis (e.g., multiple sclerosis)

Slow (Developing over Weeks to Months)
Neurosyphilis (syphilitic meningomyelitis, tabes dor-
    salis)††
Cervical spondylosis
Severe peripheral neuropathy (see 12-R)
Multiple sclerosis
Subacute combined degeneration of spinal cord††
Chronic epidural infection or granuloma (e.g., tubercu-
    lous, parasitic, fungal)
Spinal arachnoiditis††
Electrical or radiation injury
Pott's disease
Paget's disease
Ankylosing spondylitis
Polymyositis
Syringomyelia§
Amyotrophic lateral sclerosis§
Multiple cerebrovascular accidents (bilateral hemi-
    plegia)†

Childhood (or Young Adulthood) Onset†
Congenital
    Cerebral spastic diplegia
    Anomalies of spinal cord or vertebrae
Hereditary disease, e.g.:
    Werdnig-Hoffmann disease
    Muscular dystrophies
    Friedreich's ataxia
    Chronic polyneuropathies
    Niemann-Pick disease
    Tay-Sachs disease

References
1. General reference 24, p 25.
2. General reference 24, p 464.

*Except as noted, all entities may produce paralysis of either legs alone or all four extremities.
†Usually affects all four extremities.
††Usually affects legs only.
§Produces descending paralysis, or affects arms first.

12-Q. Hemiplegia (or Hemiparesis)

Cerebrovascular accident
    Thrombosis
    Embolism
    Hemorrhage
Transient ischemic attack (TIA)
Migraine syndrome
Head trauma (e.g., brain contusion, subdural or epidural
        hematoma)
Todd's paralysis
Brain tumor (primary or metastatic)
Infection (e.g., brain abscess, encephalitis, subdural em-
        pyema, meningitis)
Nonketotic hyperosmolar coma
Vasculitis

Demyelinating disease (e.g., multiple sclerosis, acute necrotizing myelitis)
Hereditary disease (e.g., leukodystrophies)
Congenital

Reference
1. General reference 24, p 25.

12-R. Peripheral Neuropathy

Primary Motor, Acute
Guillain-Barré syndrome
Infectious mononucleosis
Porphyria
Diphtheria
Hepatitis
Toxins (especially organophosphorus compounds, thallium)

Sensorimotor, Subacute
Alcoholism with associated nutritional deficiency
Beriberi
Drugs, toxins
  Arsenic
  Mercury
  Thallium
  Antimony
  Lead
  Industrial solvents
  Carbon monoxide
  Nitrofurantoin
  Vincristine
  Phenytoin
  Primidone
  Isoniazid
  Disulfiram
  Hydralazine
Diabetes mellitus
Atherosclerosis
Polyarteritis nodosa

Sarcoidosis
Subacute asymmetric idiopathic polyneuritis

Sensorimotor, Chronic
Carcinoma
Amyloidosis
Paraproteinemia (especially multiple myeloma, macro-
    globulinemia, cryoglobulinemia)
Uremia
Beriberi
Alcoholism
Diabetes mellitus
Connective-tissue disease (especially lupus)
Myxedema
Leprosy
Hereditary disease
    Charcot-Marie-Tooth disease
    Déjerine-Sottas disease
    Hereditary sensory neuropathy
    Refsum's disease
    Abetalipoproteinemia
    Tangier disease
    Metachromatic leukodystrophy
    Roussy-Lévy syndrome
    Fabry's disease
    Familial dysautonomia

Reference
1. Adams RD, Asbury AK: Diseases of the Peripheral
    Nervous System. In general reference 1, p 2027.

12-S. Carpal Tunnel Syndrome

Prolonged pressure
Trauma
Fibrosis
Tenosynovitis
Rheumatoid arthritis
Edema
Hypothyroidism
Acromegaly
Amyloidosis
Tuberculosis, other granulomatous diseases (e.g., sarcoidosis)
Gouty tophi

Reference
1. Adams RD, Asbury AK: Diseases of the Peripheral Nervous System. General reference 1, p 2027.

12-T. Cerebrospinal Fluid Characteristics in Various Diseases

Condition	Pressure	WBCs/mm³	Predominant Type of WBCs	Glucose (mg/dl)	Protein (mg/dl)	Other
Normal	7–20 cm H_2O	< 5	Lymphocytes	50–75% of serum value	< 50	
Meningitis						
Bacterial	↑	1000–20,000	85–95% neutrophils	< 40, or < 40% of blood sugar	100–500	
Viral	Normal to ↑	25–500	Sometimes neutrophils early, then lymphocytes	Normal but occasionally →	50–150	
Tuberculous	↑	50–500	Lymphocytes	< 40	100–200	
Fungal	Variably ↑	25–1000	Lymphocytes	20–40	25–500	
Syphilitic	↑	200–500	Lymphocytes	Normal	40–200	↑ globulins, positive serology

Condition	Pressure	WBCs/mm³	Predominant Type of WBCs	Glucose (mg/dl)	Protein (mg/dl)	Other
Herpes encephalitis	Normal to ↑	0–500	Lymphocytes	Normal, sometimes ↓	50–100	↑ RBCs, xanthochromia
Brain abscess	↑ – ↑↑	20–300 (may be > 50,000 if ruptured)	Neutrophils and lymphocytes	Normal	75–300	
Neoplasm	Usually ↑	< 100	Lymphocytes	40–80	50–1000	
Cerebral hemorrhage	↑ in 50%	↑ in proportion to RBCs		Normal	↑↑	↑↑ RBCs, xanthochromia
Multiple sclerosis	Normal	< 100	Lymphocytes	Normal	< 100	↑ γ globulins

References

1. General reference 24.
2. Fishman RA: Cerebrospinal Fluid. In general reference 25, vol 1, chap 5, p 1.

12-U. Dermatome Chart

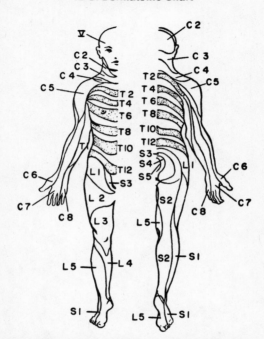

Source: Gatz AJ: *Manter's Essentials of Clinical Neuroanatomy and Neurophysiology* (4th ed). Philadelphia: Davis, 1970, p 23.

13
Respiratory System

13-A. Cough

Acute
Tracheobronchitis
Pneumonitis (see 13-G)
Lung abscess
Asthma
Pulmonary edema (see 13-L)
Gastric or other fluid aspiration
Bronchiolitis
Pulmonary thromboembolism
Inhalation of very hot or very cold air
Laryngeal inflammation or neoplasm
Foreign body in airway
Inhalation of noxious fumes
External or middle ear disease, acute

Chronic*
"Smoker's cough"
Postnasal drip (controversial)
Chronic bronchitis
Asthma
Neoplasm (usually endobronchial and malignant)
Bronchiectasis
Diffuse interstitial lung disease (see 13-O)
Chronic gastric or other fluid aspiration
Granulomatous disease (including Wegener's
    granulomatosis)

Chronic pulmonary edema
Cystic fibrosis
Pulmonary alveolar proteinosis
Mediastinal disease (e.g., aortic aneurysm)
Mesothelioma
Miscellaneous upper airway lesions (e.g., impacted cerumen in external ear)

References

1. Scadding JG: Cough. In general reference 6, p 186.
2. Tisi GM, Braunwald E: Cough and Hemoptysis. In general reference 1, p 159.
3. Irwin RS, Rosen MJ, Braman SS: Cough. *Arch Intern Med* 137:1186, 1977.

*Entities listed under "Chronic" may also present as acute cough.

13-B. Dyspnea

Acute
Pleuropulmonary causes
   Upper airway obstruction (see 13-C)
   Acute tracheobronchitis
   Foreign-body aspiration
   Pneumothorax
   Pneumonitis
   Pulmonary edema (see 13-L)
   Asthma
   Gastric or other fluid aspiration
   Pulmonary thromboembolism
   Collapse of lung segment(s)
   Pleurisy and/or pleural effusion
   Acute bronchiolitis
   Pulmonary contusion and/or flail chest
   Noxious-gas inhalation (including carbon monoxide)
Nonpulmonary causes
   Decreased pressure of inspired oxygen (e.g., at high altitude)

Acute neuromuscular dysfunction
Shock
Fever
Increased intracranial pressure
Metabolic acidosis
Psychogenic

Chronic*
Pleuropulmonary causes
    Chronic bronchitis and/or emphysema (chronic
       obstructive pulmonary disease)
    Asthma
    Bronchiectasis
    Diffuse interstitial lung disease
    Chest wall abnormalities
    Pleural disease
       Effusion
       Fibrothorax
       Primary or metastatic neoplasm
    Alveolar filling diseases
       Chronic pulmonary edema
       Alveolar cell carcinoma
       Desquamative interstitial pneumonitis
       Pulmonary alveolar proteinosis
       Alveolar microlithiasis
       Lipoid pneumonia
    Lung resection
    Paralyzed hemidiaphragm
    Upper airway obstruction
Nonpulmonary causes
    Anemia
    Obesity
    Ascites
    Hyperthyroidism
    Arteriovenous shunt
    Abnormal hemoglobin
    Psychogenic disorders

References
1. Schwarz MI, Cox PM: Dyspnea. In general reference 4,
   p 114.
2. Ingram RH, Braunwald E: Dyspnea and Pulmonary
   Edema. In general reference 1, p 162.

*Entities listed under "Chronic" may present acutely.

13-C. Wheezing

Asthma
Extrinsic
Intrinsic
Exercise-induced
Drug-induced
  Aspirin
  Beta-blockers (e.g., propranolol)
  Acetylcysteine

Wheezing of Other Etiologies
Upper airway obstruction
  Extrinsic
    Enlarged thyroid
    Lymphoma
    Edema of, or hemorrhage into, subcutaneous tissues
      of neck
    Retropharyngeal edema, hemorrhage, abscess
  Intrinsic
    Epiglottitis
    Foreign body
    Tracheal fracture, stricture, tracheomalacia
    Laryngeal tumor, trauma, edema, spasm
Large airway obstruction
  Extrinsic
    Mediastinal hemorrhage or tumor
    Vascular compression
      Aortic aneurysm
      Congenital anomalies
  Intrinsic
    Tracheal stricture, tumor, tracheomalacia
Peripheral airway obstruction
  Bronchitis, chronic and acute
  Bronchiolitis
  Bronchiectasis
  Cystic fibrosis
  Pneumonia
  Tuberculosis
Cardiac asthma
  Pulmonary edema (see 13-L)
Pulmonary embolus
Aspiration
  Foreign body
  Gastric contents
Anaphylaxis
Pulmonary infiltrates with eosinophilia

Loeffler's syndrome
Tropical eosinophilia
Chronic eosinophilic pneumonia
Bronchopulmonary aspergillosis
Polyarteritis nodosa
Irritant inhalants
Angioedema
Idiopathic
Hereditary angioneurotic edema
Carcinoid syndrome

Reference

1. MacDonnell KF: Differential Diagnosis of Asthma. In Weiss EB, Segal MS (Eds): *Bronchial Asthma: Mechanisms and Treatment.* Boston: Little, Brown, 1976, p 679.

13-D. Hemoptysis

Pseudohemoptysis

Blood of upper gastrointestinal origin
Upper airway lesions
Oropharyngeal carcinoma
Laryngeal carcinoma or other lesions
Epistaxis
Gingival bleeding
Hereditary hemorrhagic telangiectasia
Serratia marcescens infection

Tracheobronchial Sources

Tracheobronchitis
Bronchogenic carcinoma
Bronchiectasis
Foreign body
Endobronchial metastatic neoplasm
Bronchial adenoma
Traumatized bronchus
Cystic fibrosis
Broncholithiasis
Amyloidosis

Pulmonary Parenchymal Sources
Pneumonitis
Granulomatous disease including fungus balls
Lung abscess
Lung contusion or laceration
Goodpasture's syndrome
Wegener's granulomatosis
Idiopathic pulmonary hemosiderosis
Hydatid disease
Sequestration
Parasitic infestation
Pulmonary endometriosis
Neoplasm

Cardiovascular Disorders
Pulmonary thromboembolism
Pulmonary edema
Mitral stenosis
Aortic aneurysm
Primary pulmonary hypertension
Arteriovenous malformation
Eisenmenger's disease
Pulmonary vasculitis (e.g., Behçet's syndrome)
Pulmonary veno-occlusive disease

Hematologic Disorders
Coagulopathy
  Congenital
  Acquired, including anticoagulant therapy
Thrombocytopenia (see 8-P)

Undiagnosed*

References
1. Tisi GM, Braunwald E: Cough and Hemoptysis. In general reference 1, p 159.
2. Lyons HA: Differential Diagnosis of Hemoptysis and Its Treatment. *Basics of RD* 5(2), 1976.

*Five to fifteen percent despite extensive evaluation.

13-E. Cyanosis*

Central Cyanosis
Pseudocyanosis
   Polycythemia vera
   Argyria
   Hemochromatosis
Arterial desaturation
   Pulmonary disease
   Cardiac disease with right-to-left shunt
   Decreased partial pressure of inspired oxygen
Hemoglobin abnormalities
   Hemoglobin with low affinity for oxygen (e.g., hemoglobin Kansas)
   Methemoglobinemia
   Sulfhemoglobinemia

Peripheral Cyanosis
Reduced cardiac output
Arterial obstruction
Venous stasis and/or obstruction
Cold exposure (including Raynaud's phenomenon)

References
1. Braunwald E: Cyanosis, Hypoxia, and Polycythemia. In general reference 1, p 166.
2. Guenter CA: Respiratory Function of the Lungs and Blood. In Guenter CA, Welch MA (Eds): *Pulmonary Medicine*. Philadelphia: Lippincott, 1977, p 124.

*Indicates ≥5 gm of unsaturated hemoglobin or ≥1.5 gm of methemoglobin present.

13-F. Pleuritic Pain*

Chest Wall Disease
Bony thorax
  Rib fracture or tumor
  Periostitis of rib
  Periosteal hematoma
  Costochondritis (Tietze's syndrome)
  Fractured cartilage
  Xiphoidalgia
  Thoracic spondylitis due to arthritis, infection, trauma
Soft tissues
  Muscle spasm (intercostal or pectoral)
  Myositis (see 11-D)
  Fibromyositis
Neural structures
  Neurofibromatosis
  Herpes zoster
  Intercostal neuritis
  Causalgia
  Anterior chest wall syndrome

Pleural Disease
Pneumothorax
Idiopathic pleurodynia
Infectious pleuritis (see 13-H)
Immunologic disorders
  Systemic lupus erythematosus
  Rheumatoid disease
  Polyarteritis nodosa
  Progressive systemic sclerosis
  Wegener's granulomatosis
Neoplasm
  Primary
  Metastatic
Trauma
Diaphragmatic irritation
Uremic pleuritis
Post–myocardial-infarction syndrome (Dressler's syndrome)

Pulmonary Disease
Pulmonary embolism or infarction
Pneumonia
Trauma
Tumor, primary or metastatic
Middle lobe syndrome

Primary pulmonary hypertension
Fibrosing alveolitis

Mediastinal Disease
Pneumomediastinum
Mediastinitis
Pericarditis
Tumor, primary or metastatic

References
1. Reich NE, Fremont RE: *Chest Pain: Systemic Differentiation and Treatment.* New York: Macmillan, 1961.
2. General reference 5, p 224.

*Pain accentuated by breathing, coughing, or sneezing

13-G. Pneumonia*†

Bacteria
Gram-positive aerobes
  Streptococcus pneumoniae
  Staphylococcus aureus
  Strep. pyogenes
  Bacillus anthracis
  Listeria monocytogenes
Gram-negative aerobes
  Pseudomonadaceae
    Pseudomonas aeruginosa
    P. pseudomallei (melioidosis)
    P. mallei (glanders)
Enterobacteriaceae
  Klebsiella pneumoniae
  Enterobacter aeruginosa
  Serratia marcescens
  Escherichia coli
  Bacillus proteus
  Salmonella species

Infection of the lung parenchyma.
†See also 9-P

      Acinetobacter
      Providencia species
      Legionella pneumophila
   Others
      Haemophilus influenzae
      Bordetella pertussis
      Francisella tularensis
      Yersinia pestis (plague)
      Pasteurella multocida
      Brucella species
      Neisseria meningitidis
      Leptospira species
Anaerobes
Mycobacteria
   Mycobacterium tuberculosis
   M. kansasii
   M. intracellulare
   M. scrofulaceum
   M. fortuitum
Higher bacteria
   Actinomyces israelii
   Nocardia asteroides

Fungi
Histoplasma capsulatum
Coccidioides immitis
Blastomyces dermatitidis
B. brasiliensis
Cryptococcus neoformans
Candida albicans
Torulopsis glabrata
Aspergillus fumigatus
Mucormycosis
Geotrichum species
Sporotrichum schenckii

Mycoplasma pneumoniae

Viruses
Myxovirus
   Influenza virus
   Parainfluenza virus
   Respiratory syncytial virus
   Rubeola
Picornavirus
   Coxsackievirus
   ECHO virus
   Poliovirus

Rhinovirus
Reovirus
Adenovirus
Herpesvirus
  Varicella-zoster
  Variola
  Cytomegalovirus
  Epstein-Barr virus

Chlamydia
Chlamydia psittaci (psittacosis)

Rickettsiae
Coxiella burnetii (Q fever)
Rickettsia tsutsugamushi (scrub typhus)

Parasites
Protozoans
  Entamoeba histolytica
  Toxoplasma gondii
  Pneumocystis carinii
Metazoans
  Ascaris lumbricoides
  Strongyloides
  Trichinella spiralis
  Wuchereria bancrofti (filariasis)
  Pulmonary larva migrans
  Echinococcus granulosus
  Paragonimus westermani
  Schistosomiasis

Reference
1. General reference 26, p 657.

13-H. Pleural Effusion: Exudate*

Etiology	Characteristics of Exudate
Infections	
Bacterial	
Empyema (especially *Staphylococcus aureus*, gram-negative bacilli, anaerobes)	Purulent or serous
Parapneumonic (especially *Strep. pneumoniae*)	Serous
Viral	Serous
Tuberculous	Serous
Mycoplasmal	Serous
Rickettsial	Serous
Fungal (especially *Actinomyces israelii*, *Nocardia* species)	Purulent or serous
Parasitic (including *Entamoeba histolytica*, *Paragonimus westermani*, *Echinococcus granulosus*)	Serous or serofibrinous
Immunologic Disorders	
Systemic lupus erythematosus	Serous
Rheumatoid disease	Serous
Wegener's granulomatosis	Serous
Polyarteritis nodosa	Serous or serosanguineous
Progressive systemic sclerosis	Serous
Neoplasms	
Bronchogenic carcinoma	Serous or serosanguineous†
Metastatic carcinoma	Serous or serosanguineous†
Lymphoma	Serosanguineous or chylous
Mesothelioma	Bloody
Multiple myeloma	Serosanguineous

Etiology	Characteristics of Exudate
Primary chest wall neoplasm	Serosanguineous
Direct invasion of pleura, especially secondary to breast, liver, pancreatic carcinoma	Serosanguineous
Waldenström's macro-globulinemia	Serous
Ovarian neoplasm (Meigs's syndrome)	Serous†
Thromboembolic Disease	
Pulmonary embolus or in-farction	Serous or serosanguine-ous†
Inhalational Disease	
Asbestosis	Serous or serosanguine-ous
Trauma	
Open- or closed-chest	Blood (hemothorax) Chyle (chylothorax) Ingested food (ruptured esophagus)
Post-abdominal surgery	Serous
Other Causes	
Myxedema	Serous
Subphrenic abscess	Serous
Post-myocardial-infarction syndrome	Serous
Spontaneous pneumothorax	Serous
Pancreatitis	Serous or serosanguine-ous
Uremic pleuritis	Serous or serosanguine-ous
Lymphedema	Serous
Familial polyserositis	Serofibrinous
Sarcoidosis	Serous

*See also 13-K.
†Can be a transudate.

References
1. General reference 26, p 1746.
2. General reference 3, p 480.

13-I. Pleural Effusion: Transudate

Cardiac disease
  Congestive heart failure
  Constrictive pericarditis
  Obstruction of superior vena cava or azygous vein
Renal disease
  Nephrotic syndrome
  Acute glomerulonephritis
Liver disease
  Cirrhosis with ascites
Thromboembolic disease
  Pulmonary embolism*
Others
  Meigs's syndrome*
  Peritoneal dialysis
  Severe anemia
  Severe malnutrition (with hypoalbuminemia)

Reference
1. General reference 26, p 1746.

*Most are exudates.

13-J. Pleural Effusion: Exudate versus Transudate

Characteristics of an exudative effusion:

1. Pleural fluid–serum protein ratio > 0.5
2. Pleural fluid LDH > 200 IU/L
3. Pleural fluid–serum LDH ratio > 0.6

An exudate will have one or more of these three characteristics. A transudate will not have any of these characteristics.

Reference
1. Light RW, MacGregor MI, Luchsinger PC, et al: Pleural Effusions: The Diagnostic Separation of Transudates and Exudates. *Ann Intern Med* 77:507 1972.

13-K. Empyema

Pulmonary Causes
Pneumonia
Bronchial obstruction
  Tumor
  Foreign body
Hematogenous spread of infection
Bronchopleural fistula
Ruptured abscess
Spontaneous pneumothorax
Bronchiectasis
Rheumatoid disease

Mediastinal Causes
Esophageal fistula
Abscess
  Lymph node
  Osteomyelitis
Pericarditis

Subdiaphragmatic Causes
Abscess (hepatic, pancreatic, splenic, retrogastric)
Peritonitis

Direct Inoculation
Penetrating chest trauma
  Foreign body in pleural space
Iatrogenic inoculation
  Thoracentesis
  Chest tube
Postoperative
  Infected hemothorax

Leaky bronchial stump (postlobectomy or post-pneumonectomy)

Reference
1. Snider GL, Saleh SS: Empyema of the Thorax in Adults: Review of 105 Cases. *Chest* 54:410, 1968

13-L. Pulmonary Edema

Elevated Microvascular Pressure
Cardiogenic (see 2-G, ''Left Heart Failure'')
Pulmonary venous obstruction
  Chronic mediastinitis
  Anomalous pulmonary venous return
  Congenital pulmonary vein stenosis
  Idiopathic veno-occlusive disease
Volume overload (especially when associated with low plasma oncotic pressure)
Neurogenic
  Head trauma
  Intracerebral hemorrhage
  Postictal

Normal Microvascular Pressure
(Adult Respiratory Distress Syndrome)
Shock (see 2-K)
Multiple trauma
Liquid aspiration
  Gastric contents
  Water (near drowning)
  Hypertonic contrast media
  Ethyl alcohol
Acute pancreatitis
Embolism
  Fat
  Air
  Amniotic fluid
Hematologic disorders
  Diffuse intravascular coagulation

Transfusion-related leukoagglutinins
Unfiltered blood transfusion (controversial)
Infection
  Sepsis
  Pneumonia
    Bacterial
    Viral
    Mycoplasmal
    Fungal
    Pneumocystis carinii
    Legionnaires' disease
  Miliary tuberculosis
  Toxic shock syndrome
  Malaria
Inhaled toxic gases
  Oxygen (high concentration)
  Smoke
  Nitrogen dioxide
  Sulfur dioxide
  Chlorine
  Phosgene
  Ozone
  Metallic oxides
  Acid fumes
  Carbon monoxide
  Hydrocarbons
  Cadmium
  Ammonia
Associated with high negative pleural pressure
  Postthoracentesis
  Post–expansion of pneumothorax
  Acute bronchial asthma
  Complete upper airway obstruction
Pulmonary lymphatic obstruction
  Fibrotic and inflammatory disease (e.g., silicosis)
  Lymphangitic carcinomatosis
  Post–lung transplant
Miscellaneous
  Acute radiation pneumonitis
  Pulmonary contusion
  Post–cardiopulmonary bypass
  Goodpasture's syndrome
  Diabetic ketoacidosis
  Circulating vasoactive substance (e.g., histamine)
  Paraquat or Baygon
  Dextran
  Lymphangiogram dye (mechanism controversial)

Combined Elevated and Normal Microvascular Pressure

Unclear Mechanisms
High-altitude pulmonary edema
Drug overdose
   Narcotics
   Propoxyphene
   Chlordiazepoxide
   Ethchlorvynol
   Barbiturates
   Colchicine
   Aspirin

References
1. General reference 26, p 1201.
2. Ingram RH, Braunwald E: Pulmonary Edema: Cardiogenic and Noncardiogenic Forms. In general reference 8, p 571.

13-M. Respiratory Failure

Central Nervous System Disorders
Drug intoxication
   Sedatives
   Tranquilizers
   Analgesics
   Anesthetics
Vascular disorders, hypoperfusion states
   Intracranial infarction or bleeding (especially brain stem)
   Shock (see 2-K)
Trauma
   Head injury
   Increased intracranial pressure
Infection
   Viral encephalitis
   Bulbar poliomyelitis
Miscellaneous

Primary alveolar nypoventilation
Myxedema
Status epilepticus

Neuromuscular Disorders
Peripheral nerve and anterior horn cell disorders
    Guillain-Barré syndrome
    Poliomyelitis
    Amyotrophic lateral sclerosis
Myoneural junction disorders
    Myasthenia gravis
    Tetanus
    Curare-like drugs
    Anticholinesterase drugs
Muscular disorders
    Polymyositis, dermatomyositis
    Muscular dystrophies
    Myotonia
    Muscle weakness due, e.g., to hypophosphatemia
        hypokalemia

Chest Wall and Pleural Disorders
Kyphoscoliosis
Chest trauma
    Flail chest
    Multiple rib fractures
    Postthoracotomy
Pleural disorders
    Large pleural effusions (see 13-H)
    Tension pneumothorax
    Massive fibrosis

Pulmonary Disorders
Airflow limitation, chronic
    Pulmonary emphysema
    Chronic bronchitis
    Asthma, especially status asthmaticus
Airway obstruction, acute
    Foreign body
    Upper airway obstruction (see 13-C)
    Epiglottitis
    Respiratory burns
    Noxious gases
    Bronchospasm, acute (see 13-C)
Alveolar disorders
    Pneumonia
    Aspiration pneumonitis
    Pulmonary edema (see 13-L)

Elevated microvascular pressure
Normal microvascular pressure (adult respiratory distress syndrome)
Combined or unclear mechanisms
Interstitial disorders
  Fibrosing alveolitis
  Interstitial fibrosis and other diffuse disorders (see 13-O)
  Extensive neoplasm
Vascular disorders
  Pulmonary embolus (especially thrombus, fat)
  Obliterative vasculitis
    Primary pulmonary hypertension
    Scleroderma

References

1. Smith JP: Respiratory Failure and Its Management. In Holman CW, Muschenheim C (Eds): *Bronchopulmonary Diseases and Related Disorders.* New York: Harper & Row, 1972, p 694.
2. Pontoppidan H, Geffin B, and Lowenstein E: Acute Respiratory Failure. *N Engl J Med* 287:690–698, 743–752 799–806, 1972.

13-N. Obstructive Lung Disease

Chronic bronchitis
Emphysema
Asthma
Diseases associated with asthma
  Allergic bronchopulmonary aspergillosis
  Bronchocentric granulomatosis
  Mucus impaction
  Polyarteritis nodosa
Upper airway obstruction (see 13-C)
Bronchiectasis
Bronchiolitis
Interstitial lung disease (small-airways disease) (see 13-O)
Cystic fibrosis

Byssinosis
Carcinoid syndrome
Amyloidosis
Relapsing polychondritis
Chronic obstructive disease of small airways
Bronchiolitis obliterans/unilateral hyperlucent lung
(Swyer-James syndrome)
Congenital lobar emphysema
Bronchiolectasis (associated with history of irritant gas
inhalation)
Bronchiolithiasis
Sjögren's syndrome
Tracheomalacia
Kartagener's syndrome
Yellow nail syndrome
Tracheobronchopathia osteochondroplastica
Familial dysautonomia (Riley-Day syndrome)

References
1. General reference 26, p 1298.
2. Fulmer JD, Roberts WC: Small Airways and Interstitial
   Pulmonary Disease. *Chest* 77:470, 1980.

13-O. Restrictive Lung Disease

Decreased Lung Distensibility
Infection (see 13-G)
Interstitial fibrosis
    Known cause
        Environmental or occupational inhaled irritants
        Drug reaction (e.g., bleomycin, busulfan)
        Cardiac disease
        Infectious disease
        Pulmonary vascular disease
        Neoplastic disease
    Unknown cause
        Idiopathic pulmonary fibrosis
        Rheumatoid disease
        Sarcoidosis

        Scleroderma
        Systemic lupus erythematosus
        Dermatomyositis, polymyositis
        Sjögren's syndrome
        Mixed connective-tissue disease
        Ankylosing spondylitis
        Eosinophilic granuloma
        Idiopathic pulmonary hemosiderosis
        Alveolar microlithiasis
        Goodpasture's syndrome
        Familial pulmonary fibrosis
Interstitial congestion
  Left ventricular failure
  Diffuse capillary injury (adult respiratory distress syndrome)
  Pulmonary lymphatic obstruction

Replacement of Lung Parenchyma with Unventilated Tissue
Alveolar pneumonia (see 13-G)
Pulmonary edema (see 13-L)
  Elevated microvascular pressure
  Normal microvascular pressure (adult respiratory distress syndrome)
  Combined and unclear mechanisms
Atelectasis
Tumor
Sarcoidosis
Alveolar proteinosis
Amyloidosis

Lung Compression
Tumor
Pleural fluid
Fibrothorax
Pneumothorax
Cardiomegaly
Pericardial effusion

Neuromuscular Disease
Guillain-Barré syndrome
Spinal cord trauma or disease
Poliomyelitis
Amyotrophic lateral sclerosis
Myasthenia gravis
Tetanus
Polymyositis, dermatomyositis
Muscular dystrophies

Myotonia
Phrenic nerve paralysis
Other causes of muscle weakness (see 11-D)

Decreased Chest Wall Mobility
Scarring (especially secondary to burns)
Scoliosis
Kyphosis
Spondylitis
Trauma, pain
Mechanical constriction (e.g., body cast)
Scleroderma
Obesity

Reference
1. General reference 3, p 480.

13-P. Pulmonary Hypertension

Pulmonary Arterial Hypertension (Precapillary)
Vascular disease
  Increased flow
    Patent ductus arteriosus
    Atrial septal defect
      Eisenmenger physiology
    Ventricular septal defect
    Sinus of Valsalva aneurysm
  Decreased flow
    Tetralogy of Fallot
  Primary pulmonary hypertension
  Pulmonary thromboembolic disease
    Thrombotic
    Metastatic neoplasm
    Septic
    Fat
    Foreign material (e.g., talc, mercury)
    Amniotic fluid
    Parasitic (e.g., schistosomiasis)
    Primary pulmonary artery thrombosis with hemoglo-
      bin SS and SC disease

Pulmonary arteritis
    Raynaud's syndrome
    Scleroderma
    CRST syndrome
    Schistosomiasis
    Rheumatoid disease
    Systemic lupus erythematosus
    Polymyositis, dermatomyositis
    Takayasu's arteritis
    Granulomatous arteritis
Lung and pleural disease
  Emphysema
  Diffuse interstitial or alveolar disease (see 13-O)
    Sarcoidosis
    Other granulomatous diseases
    Interstitial fibrosis
    Neoplasm
      Metastatic
      Alveolar cell carcinoma
    Bronchiectasis
    Alveolar microlithiasis
    Alveolar proteinosis
    Idiopathic hemosiderosis
    Cystic fibrosis
    Post lung resection
  Pleural disease
    Fibrothorax
  Chest deformity
    Kyphoscoliosis
    Thoracoplasty
    Poliomyelitis
    Muscular dystrophy
  Alveolar hypoventilation
    Neuromuscular (see 11-D)
    Obesity
    Primary alveolar hypoventilation
    Sleep apnea-hypersomnolence syndrome
    Chronic upper airway obstruction in children
  High-altitude pulmonary hypertension

Pulmonary Venous Hypertension (Postcapillary)
Pulmonary venous disease
    Mediastinal neoplasm or granulomas
    Mediastinitis
    Anomalous pulmonary venous return
    Congenital pulmonary venous stenosis
    Idiopathic pulmonary veno-occlusive disease
Cardiac disease

Left ventricular failure (see 2-G)
Mitral valve disease (see 2-N)
    Mitral stenosis
    Mitral insufficiency
Left atrial obstruction
    Myxoma or other tumor
    Supravalvular stenotic ring
    Thrombus
Cor triatriatum

References
1. General reference 26, p 1203.
2. Fowler NO: Pulmonary Hypertension. In GE Baum (Ed): *Textbook of Pulmonary Diseases* (2nd ed). Boston: Little, Brown, 1974, p 701.
3. Moser KM (Ed): *Pulmonary Vascular Diseases.* New York: Marcel Dekker, Inc., 1979.

13-Q. Common Acute Chest Roentgenographic Infiltrates

Pseudoinfiltrate
    Poor inspiration
    Pleural effusion (free and/or loculated)
    Superimposed normal structures
Pneumonitis (any etiology)
Pulmonary infarction
Gastric or other fluid aspiration
Pulmonary edema (see 13-L)
Collapse of lung segment(s)
Pulmonary parenchymal hemorrhage (see 13-D)
Pulmonary contusion

References
1. General reference 26, p 341.
2. Felson B: *Chest Roentgenology.* Philadelphia: Saunders, 1973.

13-R. Elevated Hemidiaphragm

Pseudoelevation
Subpulmonic effusion
Diaphragmatic neoplasm

True Elevation
Paralysis or paresis due to ipsilateral phrenic nerve dysfunction
    Bronchogenic carcinoma or mediastinal malignancy
    Surgical or nonsurgical trauma
    Neurologic disorders
        Myelitis
        Encephalitis
        Herpes zoster
        Poliomyelitis
        Serum sickness following tetanus antitoxin
        Diphtheria
    Extrinsic pressure
        Substernal thyroid
        Aortic aneurysm
    Infection
        Tuberculosis
        Pneumonia
        Following empyema or pleuritis
        Following subphrenic or hepatic abscess
    Idiopathic
Intraabdominal pathology
    Subphrenic or hepatic abscess
    Other intrahepatic mass lesion, especially malignancy
    Other intraabdominal mass
    Splenic infarct
Ipsilateral lung volume loss
Pulmonary thromboembolism
Eventration

References
1. Riley EA: Idiopathic Diaphragmatic Paralysis. *Am J Med* 32:404, 1962.
2. General reference 26, p 1871.

13-S. Mediastinal Masses by Predominant Compartment

Anterior
Substernal thyroid
Thymoma
Germinal cell neoplasm (e.g., dermoid)
Lymphoma
Ascending aortic aneurysm
Parathyroid tumor
Mesenchymal neoplasm (e.g., lipoma or fibroma)
Hematoma

Middle
Lymphoma
Metastatic neoplasm (pulmonary or extrapulmonary)
Sarcoidosis
Infectious granulomatous disease
Bronchogenic cyst
Vascular dilatation
Aortic arch aneurysm
Vascular anomaly
Lymph node hyperplasia
Infectious mononucleosis
Primary or tracheal neoplasm
Hematoma

Anterior Cardiophrenic Angle
Pleuropericardial cyst or tumor
Foramen of Morgagni hernia
Fat pad
Diaphragmatic lymph node enlargement (e.g., lymphoma)
Pulmonary parenchymal mass
Cardiac aneurysm
Pericardial fat necrosis

Posterior
Neurogenic tumor
Meningocele
Esophageal lesion
  Neoplasm
  Diverticulum
  Megaesophagus of any etiology (e.g., achalasia)
  Hiatus hernia
  Bochdalek hernia
Thoracic spine lesion
  Neoplasm

    Infectious spondylitis
    Fracture with hematoma
    Extramedullary hematopoiesis
Descending aortic aneurysm
Mediastinal abscess
Pancreatic pseudocyst
Lymph node hyperplasia
Hematoma
Cystic lesion
    Neurenteric cyst
    Gastroenteric cyst
    Thoracic duct

References
1. General reference 26, p 1793.
2. Wychulis AR, Payne WS, Clagett OT, et al: Surgical Treatment of Mediastinal Tumors: A 40 Year Experience. *J Thorac Cardiovasc Surg* 62:379, 1971.

13-T. Pulmonary Risk Factors for Thoracic and Abdominal Surgery

Significant smoking history
Obesity
Age >60 years
Severe intercurrent disease
Arterial blood gases
    Arterial PCO_2 > 45 mmHg
    Hypoxemia not reliable
Spirometry
    Forced vital capacity < 50% of predicted
    Forced expiratory volume in 1 sec < 2.0 L
    Maximal ventilatory volume < 50% of predicted

References
1. Tisi G: State of the Art: Preoperative Evaluation of Pulmonary Function. *Am Rev Respir Dis* 119:295, 1979.
2. Epstein PE: Preoperative Evaluation of the Patient with Pulmonary Disease. In AP Fishman (Ed): *Pulmonary Diseases and Disorders.* New York: McGraw-Hill, 1980, p 1645.

General References

1. Isselbacher KJ, Adams RD, Braunwald E, et al (Eds): *Harrison's Principles of Internal Medicine* (9th ed). New York: McGraw-Hill, 1980.
2. Freitag JJ, Miller LW (Eds): *Manual of Medical Therapeutics* (23rd ed). Boston: Little, Brown, 1980.
3. Harvey AM, Bordley J, Barondess JA: *Differential Diagnosis: The Interpretation of Clinical Evidence* (3rd ed). Philadelphia: Saunders, 1979.
4. Friedman HH (Ed): *Problem-Oriented Medical Diagnosis* (2nd ed). Boston: Little, Brown, 1979.
5. DeGowin EL, DeGowin RL: *Bedside Diagnostic Examination* (3rd ed). New York: Macmillan, 1976.
6. Hart FD (Ed): *French's Index of Differential Diagnosis* (11th ed). Bristol, England: John Wright & Sons Ltd., 1979.

Acid-Base and Electrolyte Disorders
7. Maxwell MH, Kleeman CR (Eds): *Clinical Disorders of Fluid and Electrolyte Metabolism.* New York: McGraw-Hill, 1980.

Cardiovascular System
8. Braunwald E (Ed): *Heart Disease: A Textbook of Cardiovascular Medicine.* Philadelphia: Saunders, 1980.

Endocrine/Metabolic System
9. Bondy PK, Rosenberg LE: *Metabolic Control and Disease* (8th ed). Philadelphia: Saunders, 1980.
10. Williams RH (Ed): *Textbook of Endocrinology* (5th ed). Philadelphia: Saunders, 1974.

Eye
11. Newell FW, Ernest JT: *Ophthalmology* (3rd ed). St. Louis: Mosby, 1974.
12. Scheie HG, Albert DM: *Textbook of Ophthalmology* (9th ed). Philadelphia: Saunders, 1977.

Gastrointestinal and Hepatic Systems
13. Bockus HL (Ed): *Gastroenterology* (3rd ed). Philadelphia: Saunders, 1974.
14. Schiff L (Ed): *Diseases of the Liver* (4th ed). Philadelphia: Lippincott, 1975.
15. Sleisenger MH, Fordtran JS: *Gastrointestinal Disease* (2nd ed). Philadelphia: Saunders, 1978.

Genitourinary System
16. Brenner BM, Rector FC (Eds): *The Kidney* (2nd ed). Philadelphia: Saunders, 1981.
17. Schrier RW (Ed): *Renal and Electrolyte Disorders* (2nd ed). Boston: Little, Brown, 1980.
18. Earley LW, Gottschalk CW (Eds): *Strauss and Welt's Diseases of the Kidney* (3rd ed). Boston: Little, Brown, 1979.

Hematologic System
19. Miale JB: *Laboratory Medicine: Hematology* (5th ed). St. Louis: Mosby, 1977.
20. Williams WJ, Beutler E, Erslev AJ, et al (Eds): *Hematology* (2nd ed). New York: McGraw-Hill, 1977.

Infectious Disease
21. Mandell GL, Douglas RG, Bennett JE (Eds): *Principles and Practice of Infectious Diseases.* New York: Wiley, 1979.

Integument
22. Fitzpatrick TB, Eisen AZ, Wolff K, et al (Eds): *Dermatology in General Medicine* (2nd ed). New York: McGraw-Hill, 1979.

Musculoskeletal System
23. McCarty DJ (Ed): *Arthritis and Allied Conditions: A Textbook of Rheumatology* (9th ed). Philadelphia: Lea & Febiger, 1979.

Nervous System

24. Adams RD, Victor M: *Principles of Neurology.* New York: McGraw-Hill, 1977.
25. Baker AB, Baker LH (Eds): *Clinical Neurology.* New York: Harper & Row, 1980.

Respiratory System

26. Fraser RG, Paré JAP (Eds): *Diagnosis of Diseases of the Chest* (2nd ed). Philadelphia: Saunders, 1978.

Index